RENAL DIET COOKBOOK FOR SENIORS

Quick and Easy Mouthwatering Recipes for Kidney Health

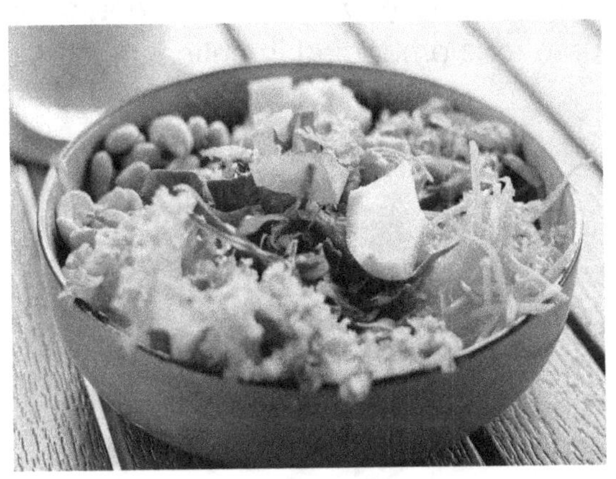

LYNNE Q. CHAPMAN

TABLE OF CONTENTS

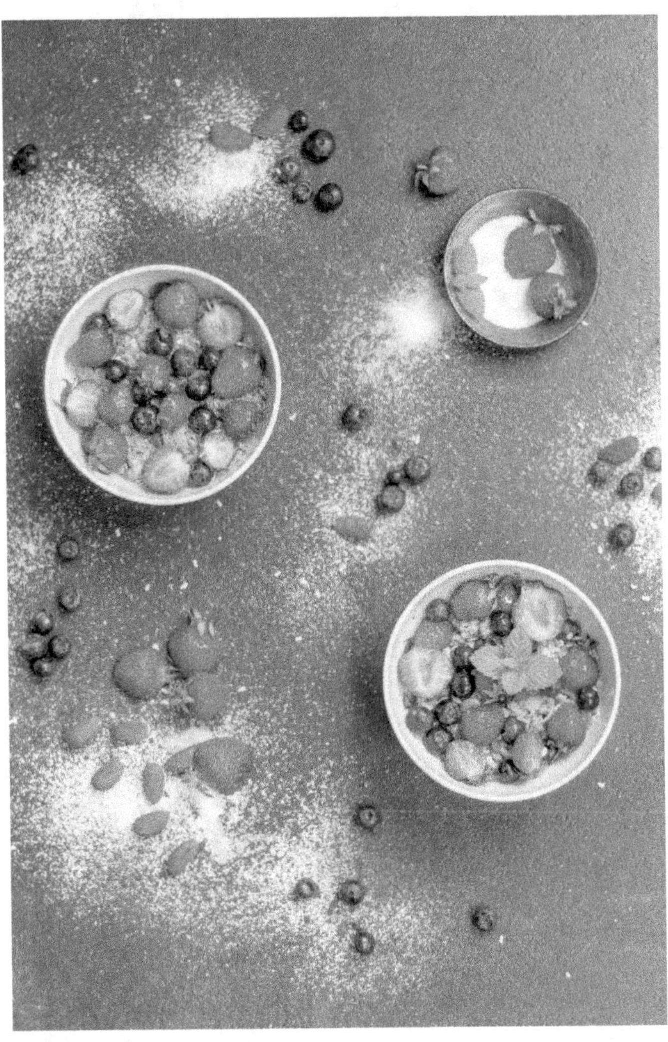

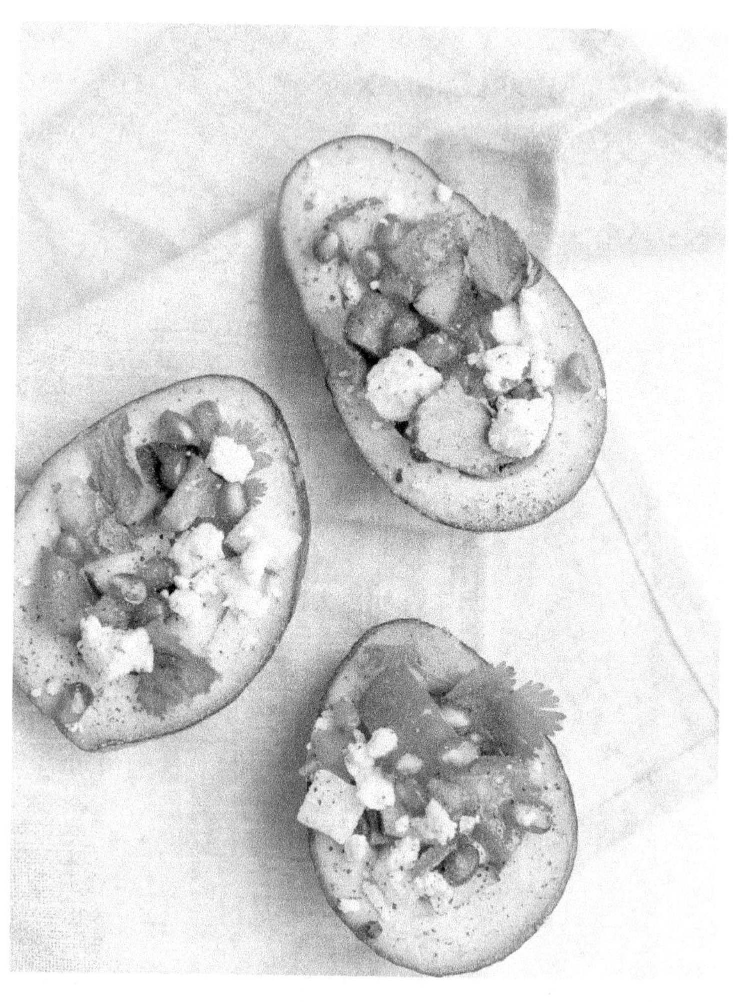

INTRODUCTION

As we age, the risk of kidney and urinary tract diseases increases; our bodies go through a lot of changes, and our dietary needs change too. So, it is essential to be aware of the age-related changes in kidney function and the potential impact on overall health. According to the Better Health Channel, older individuals are more susceptible to kidney and urinary tract problems, and conditions such as diabetes, high blood pressure, obesity, and heart disease can further elevate the risk. Chronic kidney disease (CKD) is a common concern in the elderly, often associated with comorbidities like hypertension and diabetes.

For seniors, maintaining a healthy diet is crucial to prevent or manage chronic conditions such as kidney disease. Unfortunately, many seniors struggle to find delicious and nutritious meals that fit their dietary restrictions. That's where the Renal Diet Cookbook for Seniors comes to play.

Imagine your loved one, a senior who has been diagnosed with kidney disease, feeling overwhelmed and confused about what they can and cannot eat. They may feel like they have to give up all their favorite foods and flavors, leading to a sense of loss and isolation. But with this Renal Diet Cookbook for Seniors, they can enjoy a wide variety of tasty and satisfying meals that are tailored to their specific dietary needs.

This cookbook is not just a collection of recipes, but a comprehensive guide to understanding the renal diet and how it can benefit seniors with kidney disease. It includes tips on meal planning, grocery shopping, and cooking techniques that make it easy to follow the diet without sacrificing flavor or variety. Each recipe is carefully crafted to meet the nutritional requirements of seniors with kidney disease, while still being delicious and easy to prepare.

The Renal Diet Cookbook for Seniors is more than just a cookbook. It's a tool for seniors and their caregivers to take control of their health and well-being. By following the recipes and guidelines in this cookbook, seniors can improve their kidney function, reduce their risk of complications, and enjoy a better quality of life.

Understanding Renal Health in Seniors

As individuals age, their kidneys can be affected by various diseases and conditions, making them more susceptible to kidney and urinary tract problems. Some factors that increase the risk of kidney disease in seniors include:

- Being over 60 years of age
- Having diabetes
- Being obese
- Having high blood pressure
- Having established heart problems or a history of heart attack
- Smoking

Age-related kidney disease can lead to increased morbidity and mortality. The aging process affects the kidneys' structural and functional properties, leading to a gradual decline in glomerular filtration rate (GFR) and renal blood flow. This age-related decline in kidney function can predispose seniors to acute kidney injury and progressive chronic kidney disease. Common kidney and bladder issues in seniors include bladder control problems, urinary tract infections, and chronic kidney disease. It's crucial for seniors to be proactive about their renal health by having regular check-ups and monitoring kidney function. Early detection and proper management can significantly impact the longevity of the kidneys.

The decision to initiate renal replacement therapy (RRT) in the elderly is complex due to various challenges, including comorbid conditions and nonmedical barriers.

Understanding the physiological changes in the aging kidney is vital for providing appropriate nephrology care to elderly CKD patients.

In summary, as we age, it's important to be mindful of the changes in kidney function and the associated risks. By staying informed and proactive, seniors can take steps to preserve their renal health and overall well-being

The Importance of Diet in Renal Health

Maintaining a healthy diet is crucial for individuals with renal health issues. A renal diet can help slow kidney damage and improve overall health. A renal diet is often low in sodium, phosphorus, and sometimes potassium and protein. Sodium and potassium are minerals that help maintain fluid balance in the bloodstream and cells, and keep our nerves and muscles functioning. Eating fresh foods and cooking from scratch as much as possible is recommended, while fast food and packaged foods should be avoided due to their high sodium content. Spices and fresh or dried herbs can be used instead of salt to flavor food, and canned beans and vegetables should be rinsed before cooking to remove excess salt. Protein serving sizes should be kept small, with a serving size of protein being 2 to 3 ounces of chicken, fish, or meat.

Alcohol should be limited if not completely avoided. Keeping track of liquid intake is also important, as is understanding and keeping track of lab reports to make healthy food choices.

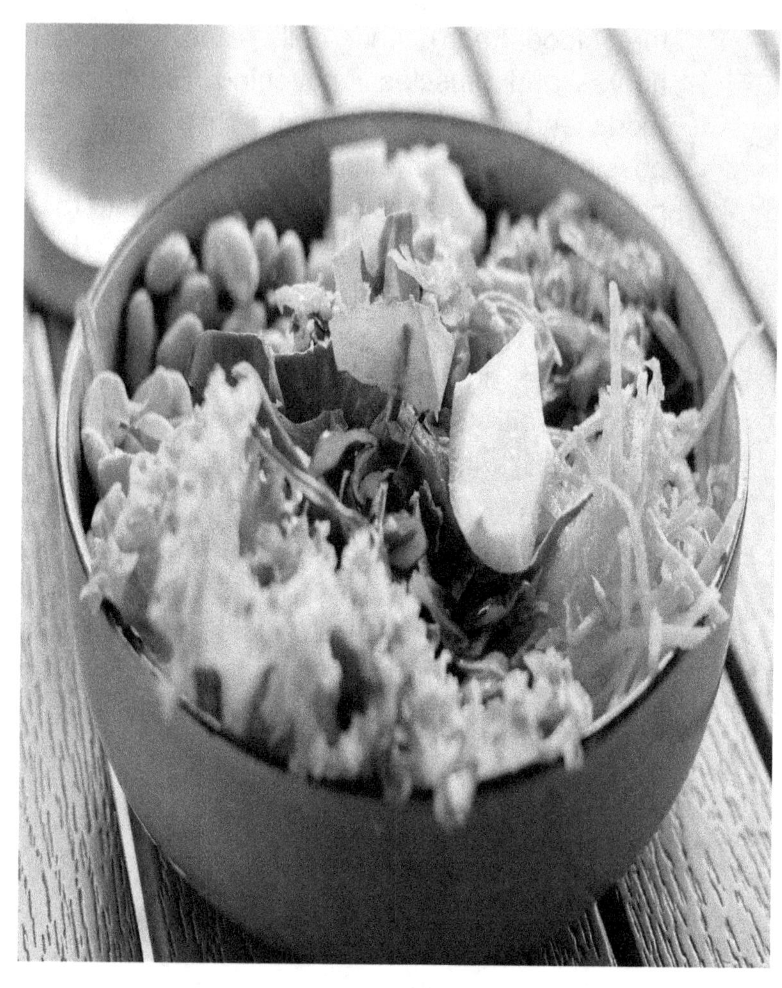

CHAPTER ONE

BASICS OF RENAL DIET

An Overview of Renal Diet

A renal diet is a special eating plan for people with kidney disease. It focuses on managing the intake of certain nutrients to help protect the kidneys and prevent further damage. Embarking on the journey of renal health involves understanding and embracing the principles of a renal diet – a tailored approach that supports the well-being of our kidneys.

The key principles of a renal diet include limiting sodium, phosphorus, potassium and protein, as well as controlling fluid intake.

Sodium Moderation:
Sodium is a mineral found in salt and is widely used to prepare foods. Sodium can tip the scales unfavorably for kidney health. A renal

diet limits and advocates for sodium moderation, helping to curb and manage excess sodium intake that might otherwise strain the kidneys and elevate blood pressure. This means reducing the consumption of salty foods and processed products, and using alternative seasonings like herbs and spices.

Phosphorus Moderation:
Phosphorus is a mineral found in many foods and can be harmful when its levels are too high in the body.
A renal diet limits phosphorus to protect the bones and blood vessels from damage. This involves avoiding high-phosphorus foods like dairy, whole grains, and certain types of meat and beans.

Potassium Moderation:
Potassium is a mineral that helps muscles work properly, but when the kidneys are not functioning well, potassium can build up in the blood and cause heart problems. Foods that are high in potassium include bananas, oranges, tomatoes, potatoes, and dairy products. Thus, a renal limits potassium intake to help protect the heart.

Protein Management:
While Protein is essential for the body, excessive amounts of it can burden or put a strain on the kidneys.
A renal diet involves controlling the amount of high-quality protein consumed to reduce the workload on the kidneys. This includes monitoring portion sizes and choosing lean sources of protein.

Mindful Fluids Intake:
A renal diet encourages a mindful approach to fluid intake, ensuring you neither flood nor deprive your kidneys. This may also involve restricting fluids to maintain a healthy balance in the body and prevent strain on the heart and lungs.
This balance is crucial in maintaining optimal hydration without overburdening these vital organs.
Managing fluid intake is important for people with kidney disease, especially those on dialysis.

Overall, a renal diet is a specialized eating plan that focuses on managing the intake of certain nutrients to protect the kidneys and prevent further damage. By following the principles of a renal diet, people with kidney disease can improve their overall health and quality of life.

Benefits Of Renal Diet

A renal diet can significantly benefit seniors with kidney disease by helping them manage their condition, slow down the progression of the disease, and prevent or manage other health complications. The benefits of a renal diet include:

Reducing the Risk of Losing Kidney Function: A renal diet is tailored to the specific needs of seniors with kidney disease, ensuring that their kidneys can function optimally.

Slowing Down Disease Progression: By following a renal diet, seniors can maintain a healthy balance of nutrients in their bodies, which can help slow down the damage to their kidneys.

Managing Other Health Complications: A renal diet can help prevent or manage other serious health problems, such as high blood pressure, heart disease, and diabetes.

Improving Overall Health: A renal diet focuses on consuming fresh fruits, vegetables, whole grains, low-fat dairy, and lean proteins, which can lead to better overall health and well-being.

Balancing Salts and Minerals: As seniors with kidney disease have impaired kidney function, they need to be cautious about their intake of sodium, potassium, and phosphorus. A renal diet helps maintain a healthy balance of these minerals in the body.

Preventing Waste Buildup: A kidney-friendly diet helps prevent the buildup of certain minerals in the body, which can cause further damage to the kidneys.

Customization: Dietitians can help seniors create a kidney-friendly eating plan that includes the foods they enjoy, accommodating special dietary preferences and restrictions.

Meal Planning and Nutrition Education: Working with a dietitian or following a comprehensive guide like the Renal Diet Cookbook for Seniors can provide valuable information on meal planning, grocery shopping, and cooking techniques, making it easier for seniors to adhere to the renal diet.

In conclusion, a renal diet is a powerful tool for seniors with kidney disease to manage their condition, improve their overall health, and maintain their quality of life. By following a renal diet, they can take control of their health and slow down the progression of kidney disease.

Common Renal Conditions in Seniors

As people age, they become more susceptible to various renal conditions that can significantly impact their quality of life. Some common renal conditions in seniors include:

Inflammation or Swelling of the Kidneys: This can be caused by conditions such as glomerulonephritis. Symptoms include blood in the urine, foamy urine, swelling in the legs, and high blood pressure

Diabetes: This is the most common cause of kidney disease in Australia and can lead to kidney failure if left untreated. Symptoms include frequent urination, fatigue, and swelling in the legs.

Urinary Tract Infections: If left untreated, these infections may spread into the kidneys.

Symptoms include pain or burning while urinating, a tendency to urinate frequently, and murky or strong-smelling urine.

High Blood Pressure: This can increase the risk of heart attack, stroke, and loss of vision, as well as cause kidney damage. Symptoms include headaches, shortness of breath, and chest pain.

Hereditary Kidney Diseases: Conditions like polycystic kidney disease can affect older individuals. Symptoms include pain in the back or side, blood in the urine, and high blood pressure.

Chronic Kidney Disease: This is defined by an estimated glomerular filtration rate (eGFR) of less than 60 mL/min/m² and is common in elderly patients.

The risk factors for kidney disease in seniors include high blood pressure, diabetes, kidney stones, a family history of kidney failure, prolonged use of over-the-counter pain medications, and being over the age of 60.

Early detection and proper treatment can increase the life of your kidneys and improve your overall health. It is essential to have regular check-ups with your doctor and ask for your kidney function to be checked. Treatment options depend on the specific condition and may include medication, lifestyle changes, and in severe cases, dialysis or kidney transplant.

Chronic Kidney Disease (CKD) Explained

Chronic Kidney Disease (CKD), in layman's terms, is a prolonged condition where the kidneys gradually lose their ability to function optimally over time.

Think of the kidneys as diligent filters that sift through the blood, removing waste and excess fluids. When CKD sets in, this intricate filtering process becomes compromised, affecting the balance of essential substances in the body.

Thus, it is a condition where the kidneys are damaged and cannot filter blood as effectively as they should. This leads to a buildup of excess fluid and waste in the body, which can cause other health problems such as heart disease and stroke. CKD can also lead to anemia, increased risk of infections, and imbalances in important minerals in the blood. It is a serious condition that usually worsens over time, but treatment can help slow down its progression. If left untreated, CKD can progress to kidney failure, requiring dialysis or a kidney transplant for survival.

Five Stages of Chronic Kidney Disease (CKD)

CKD is classified into five stages based on the level of kidney function. These stages reflect the level of impairment in kidney function and help in understanding the severity of the condition and guide treatment decisions. In the early stages, symptoms might be subtle or nonexistent, making regular check-ups crucial for early detection. As CKD advances, symptoms like fatigue, swelling, difficulty concentrating and changes in urination patterns may manifest.
The stages are as follows:

Stage 1: This stage involves kidney damage with a normal or increased Glomerular Filtration Rate (GFR) of greater than 90 mL/min/1.73 m^2. At this stage, the kidneys are still functioning well, and individuals may not experience any symptoms. However, there may be signs of kidney damage, such as the presence of protein in the urine.

Stage 2: In this stage, there is a mild reduction in GFR, ranging from 60 to 89 mL/min/1.73

m^2. Similar to stage 1, individuals may not have noticeable symptoms, but there is still evidence of kidney damage.

Stage 3: Stage 3 is further divided into two sub-stages:
- **Stage 3a:** Involves a moderate reduction in GFR, ranging from 45 to 59 mL/min/1.73 m^2.
- **Stage 3b:** Also characterized by a moderate reduction in GFR, ranging from 30 to 44 mL/min/1.73 m^2. At these stages, the reduction in kidney function may start to manifest as symptoms, and medical intervention becomes increasingly important

Stage 4: This stage is marked by a severe reduction in GFR, ranging from 15 to 29 mL/min/1.73 m^2. At this point, the kidneys are significantly impaired, and the risk of complications is higher. Treatment aims to halt the progression of the disease and control symptoms.

Stage 5: Also known as kidney failure, this stage is characterized by a GFR of less than 15 mL/min/1.73 m^2 or the need for dialysis. At this advanced stage, the kidneys are no longer able to function effectively, and treatment options may include dialysis or kidney transplantation.

These stages provide a framework for healthcare professionals to assess the progression of CKD and tailor treatment plans to each patient's specific needs. Early detection and management are crucial in slowing the progression of the disease and reducing the risk of complications.

Factors that Contributes to Chronic Kidney Disease

Various factors contribute to CKD, with hypertension, heart disease, history of kidney failure and diabetes topping the list.
These conditions are silent architects, which gradually exerts pressure on the kidneys over time. The disease is also often as a result of a combination of physical, environmental, and social factors. Other culprits include certain medications, genetic predispositions, and recurrent kidney infections. Lifestyle choices, like a diet high in sodium and low in water intake, can also play a role. Many people with CKD do not experience symptoms until the later stages, making early detection important. Thus, early detection and management are key to managing CKD.

How to Prevent CKD

CKD is a prevalent condition, with more than one in seven American adults estimated to have it. Early detection and management are crucial in slowing down the progression of the disease and preventing complications. To prevent CKD and reduce the risk of kidney failure, it is essential to control risk factors, get tested regularly, make lifestyle changes, take prescribed medication, and have regular check-ups with a healthcare provider. Managing CKD involves controlling blood pressure, eating the right foods, and following a treatment plan tailored to the underlying cause of the disease.

Managing Hypertension and Diabetes

Hypertension and diabetes often coexist in seniors, and their combination can substantially promote cardiovascular disease and chronic kidney disease. In seniors with diabetes, it is crucial to control blood pressure to prevent these complications. According to the Centers for Disease Control and Prevention, up to 67% of people aged 20 years or older with self-reported diabetes also have hypertension.

Navigating the intricate landscape of managing hypertension and diabetes in seniors requires a proactive and personalized approach. Below are key strategies to blending medical insights with practical guidance for optimal health in your senior years.

Hypertension Management: Hypertension, or elevated blood pressure, underscores the importance of maintaining vascular health, especially as we age. Blood vessels are like the thoroughfares of the circulatory system. Managing hypertension involves a multi-faceted approach. Lifestyle modifications, including a controlled sodium intake, regular physical activity, and potential pharmacological interventions, are integral. This orchestration aims to mitigate the strain on the cardiovascular system, promoting overall well-being.

Diabetes Management: Diabetes, a metabolic intricacy, demands meticulous control to safeguard various organ systems, notably the kidneys. Senior individuals with diabetes should embrace a balanced diet, emphasizing complex carbohydrates and lean proteins. Regular blood glucose monitoring, adherence to prescribed medications, and a commitment to regular exercise form the pillars of effective diabetes management. Think of these measures as a tailored regimen to maintain glycemic harmony, minimizing the risk of complications.

Lifestyle Adjustments: Lifestyle adjustments are akin to fine-tuning the engine of your health. Adopting a heart-healthy diet, characterized by fruits, vegetables, and whole grains, contributes to blood pressure and blood sugar control. Engaging in regular physical activity not only enhances cardiovascular fitness but also aids in weight management and insulin sensitivity. These choices empower seniors to actively participate in their health management, fostering a sense of control and well-being.

Regular Check-ups and Healthcare Collaboration: Regular medical check-ups are akin to routine diagnostics for your body's intricate machinery. They provide a means of early detection and intervention. Collaborating closely with healthcare professionals ensures a tailored and responsive approach to your unique health profile. Open communication about lifestyle, medication adherence, and any emerging concerns facilitates a comprehensive management plan, promoting synergy between patient and healthcare provider.

In summary, managing hypertension and diabetes in seniors requires a tailored approach that considers the specific needs and conditions of the individual. Controlling blood pressure is crucial for preventing cardiovascular and kidney complications in seniors with diabetes, and the treatment should be personalized to ensure the best possible outcomes.This proactive journey is about optimizing health, fostering resilience, and enhancing the quality of life in the golden years. By embracing these strategies, seniors can navigate the complexities of chronic conditions with informed choices and a commitment to holistic well-being.

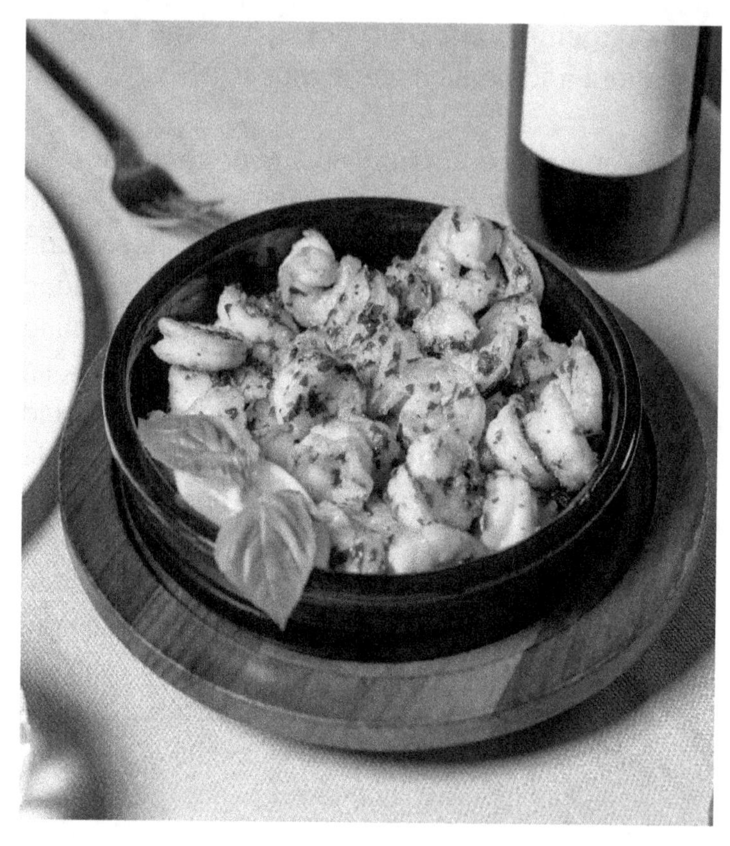

CHAPTER TWO

NUTRITIONAL REQUIREMENTS FOR SENIORS

What to Eat and Limit in a Renal Diet

Here's a guide on what to eat in a renal diet tailored for seniors:

Low-Potassium Fruits:
   - Choose fruits such as apples, berries, grapes, and peaches.
   - Limit high-potassium fruits like bananas, oranges, and melons.

Cooked Vegetables:
   - Opt for cooked vegetables like green beans, cauliflower, and carrots.
   - Limit high-potassium vegetables such as tomatoes, potatoes, and spinach.

Lean Protein Sources:

- Include lean proteins like chicken, turkey, fish, and eggs.
- Limit red meats and processed meats to control protein intake.

Low-Phosphorus Dairy:

- Choose low-phosphorus dairy options like milk, yogurt, and cheese.
- Control portions to manage phosphorus levels.

Whole Grains:

- Select whole grains like brown rice, quinoa, bulgur, and whole wheat bread.
- These provide fiber and essential nutrients without excess phosphorus.

Healthy Fats:

- Incorporate healthy fats from sources like olive oil, avocados, and nuts into your diet.
- Limit saturated and trans fats found in processed foods.

Hydration with Water:

- Stay well-hydrated with water to support kidney function.
- Limit caffeinated and sugary beverages, which may contribute to dehydration.

Herbs and Spices for Flavor:
- Use herbs and spices like garlic, basil, and lemon to add flavor without excess salt.
- Limit salt intake to manage sodium levels.

Homemade Meals:
- Prepare homemade meals to have better control over ingredients.
- This allows customization to meet specific dietary needs and preferences.

Limit Processed and Packaged Foods:
- Minimize processed and packaged foods, as they often contain hidden sodium and phosphorus.
- Opt for fresh, whole foods for better nutritional control.

Portion Control:
- Pay attention to portion sizes to avoid overloading the kidneys.
- Smaller and more frequent meals can be easier on the digestive system.

Regular Check-ups and Consultation:
- Schedule regular visits for check-ups with healthcare professionals.

- Consult with a registered dietitian to create a personalized renal diet plan tailored to specific health conditions.

Cooking Techniques for Nutrient Preservation

Several cooking techniques can be employed to preserve the nutritional value of foods in a renal diet for seniors. When preparing fish, steaming and gas oven-baking have been found to decrease phosphorus content, making them suitable methods for renal patients. Similarly, a study on legumes revealed that soaking and cooking dried and canned legumes can reduce their potassium and phosphorus content, making them more compatible with a renal diet.

In general, the following cooking techniques can help preserve the nutritional value of foods for seniors with renal issues:

Steaming: Steaming is a gentle cooking method that minimizes nutrient loss. It involves cooking food over boiling water, which helps preserve the natural flavor, texture, color, and nutrients of vegetables, fish, and poultry.

Baking: Gas oven-baking, in particular, has been shown to decrease phosphorus content in fish, making it a suitable technique for renal patients.

Soaking and Cooking Legumes: This process can reduce the potassium and phosphorus content of legumes, making them more kidney-friendly.

Boiling: Boiling is a simple technique that can be kidney-friendly if done correctly. When boiling vegetables, using minimal water and avoiding overcooking can help preserve their nutritional value. So, use minimal water, and consider using the water for soups or sauces to retain any nutrients that leach into it.

Grilling or Broiling: These methods are suitable for lean proteins like chicken, meat or fish, as they allow excess fat to drip away, preserving the protein content. They are quick cooking methods that add a smoky flavor without excessive added fats.

Poaching: Poaching involves gently simmering food in liquid, preserving the delicate texture of proteins like fish or chicken.

Use a flavorful broth or low-sodium liquid for added taste.

Roasting: Roasting allows for the use of herbs and spices to enhance flavor without relying on excessive salt. These methods are suitable for vegetables, whole grains, and lean meats.

Stir-Frying: Stir-frying involves quickly cooking small, uniform pieces of food in a small amount of oil. It's a fast method that retains the color and nutrients of vegetables, but be mindful of the oil amount.

Microwaving: Microwaving is a convenient method that preserves nutrients due to its shorter cooking times. It's suitable for cooking vegetables, grains, and proteins.

Using Herbs and Spices: Enhance the flavor of your dishes with herbs and spices instead of relying on excessive salt. Fresh or dried herbs like basil, rosemary, and thyme can add depth without compromising kidney health.

Limiting Phosphorus-Rich Ingredients: For individuals with kidney issues, limiting high-phosphorus ingredients like dairy and nuts during cooking helps manage phosphorus levels.

Monitoring Sodium Intake: Be mindful of sodium content in cooking. Opt for low-sodium broths, sauces, and seasonings to control salt intake without sacrificing taste.

Using Citrus for Flavor: Citrus fruits like lemon or lime can add a burst of flavor to dishes without relying on salt. Use them in marinades, dressings, or as a finishing touch.

Preserving Water-Soluble Vitamins: Retain water-soluble vitamins by using minimal water when cooking, and consider reserving cooking liquid for soups or sauces.

By incorporating these cooking techniques, individuals on a renal diet can enjoy flavorful meals while preserving essential nutrients. It is also important to note that the specific cooking techniques and their impact on the nutritional composition of foods may vary.

Tips on Meal Planning

Meal planning for seniors on a renal diet demands a thoughtful and strategic approach to ensure optimal nutrition while managing kidney health. By adopting a systematic and considerate planning process, seniors can enjoy a varied and satisfying diet that aligns with the dietary restrictions associated with renal conditions. Here are key tips for effective meal planning in this context:

Portion Control and Balanced Meals:

Emphasize portion control to maintain a healthy weight and reduce the workload on the kidneys. Ensure meals are balanced, comprising appropriate amounts of lean proteins, low-phosphorus grains, and a variety of colorful, low-potassium vegetables.

Selecting Kidney-Friendly Proteins:

Choose lean protein sources such as poultry, fish, eggs, and tofu while moderating intake to manage phosphorus levels. Incorporate plant-based proteins like beans and legumes as alternatives to animal proteins.

Mindful Sodium Management:

Adopt a conscious approach to sodium intake by using herbs, spices, and low-sodium alternatives to flavor meals. This helps manage blood pressure and mitigates potential complications associated with excessive sodium consumption.

Varied and Colorful Vegetables:
Incorporate a spectrum of low-potassium vegetables into meals for added nutrients and flavor. Rotate vegetables to ensure a diverse range of vitamins and minerals, supporting overall health.

Fruit Selection and Moderation:
Choose lower-potassium fruits such as apples, berries, and grapes. Practice moderation to control potassium intake while still enjoying the natural sweetness and nutritional benefits of fruits.

Hydration Prioritization:
Encourage seniors to maintain adequate hydration, as water plays a pivotal role in kidney function. Keep water easily accessible and consider incorporating hydrating foods like watermelon and cucumbers into meals.

Customized Meal Plans:
Tailor meal plans to individual preferences and dietary restrictions, ensuring seniors find enjoyment in their meals while adhering to renal guidelines. Flexibility and variety are key components of a sustainable and satisfying

meal plan. Thankfully, this is your go to cookbook which has all that you need.

In conclusion, meal planning for seniors on a renal diet demands a blend of professional guidance, awareness of nutrient content, and a commitment to variety. By adhering to these tips, seniors can embrace a renal-friendly meal plan that not only supports kidney health but also contributes to overall well-being and enjoyment of meals.

Stocking a Kidney Friendly Pantry

Creating a kidney-friendly pantry is a strategic and empowering step towards maintaining optimal renal health. By thoughtfully selecting and stocking your pantry with nutrient-rich, kidney-supportive options, you can proactively contribute to the overall well-being of your kidneys. Stocking a kidney-friendly pantry involves selecting foods that are low in sodium, potassium, and phosphorus, as well as avoiding added salt and other hidden sources of sodium. Here are some guidelines and food suggestions to help you create a kidney-friendly pantry:

Whole Grains

Incorporate whole grains such as brown rice, barley, buckwheat, bulgur, couscous, oatmeal, wild rice quinoa, and whole wheat pasta into your pantry. These grains are not only rich in fiber but also provide a steady source of energy without burdening the kidneys with excessive phosphorus.

Low-Sodium Broths and Soups

Opt for low-sodium or homemade broths and soups as flavorful bases for meals. Controlling sodium intake is paramount for kidney health, and these alternatives allow you to savor delicious dishes without compromising on dietary restrictions.

Canned Vegetables and Fruits

Stock up on low-sodium canned vegetables and fruits to ensure a convenient and kidney-friendly option. Opt for low-sodium or no-salt options, and rinse canned goods to reduce sodium content. Be cautious of hidden sources of added phosphorus and enjoy the convenience of having nutritious ingredients readily available for meals

Lean Proteins

Include lean protein sources in your pantry, such as canned tuna, skinless poultry, tofu, unsalted nuts or seeds, nut butters, and no added salt canned beans like chickpeas or lentils. These protein options are essential for muscle maintenance without exacerbating kidney stress. Be mindful of portion sizes to strike a balance in your nutritional intake.

Healthy Cooking Oils

Choose heart-healthy oils like olive oil and canola oil for your pantry. These oils are rich in monounsaturated fats and can be instrumental in supporting cardiovascular health—a key consideration for those managing kidney conditions.

Herbs and Spices

Enhance the flavor of your meals with herbs and spices instead of relying on salt. This not only adds variety to your dishes but also helps control sodium intake, a critical aspect of kidney-friendly nutrition.

Snack Smartly

Opt for kidney-friendly snacks, such as unsalted nuts, seeds, and air-popped popcorn. These snacks provide a satisfying crunch without compromising your dietary goals.

Comparing Brands: Sodium and potassium levels can vary significantly from one brand to another, so always compare labels to find the lowest sodium options.

Sauces and Condiments: Choose low-sodium (less than 140 mg per serving) or no-salt options

In summary, stocking a kidney-friendly pantry involves making informed and health-conscious choices. By incorporating these items into your pantry, you can create a foundation for nourishing, kidney-supportive meals. This proactive approach not only aligns with dietary recommendations for renal health but also empowers you to enjoy a varied and flavorful diet while prioritizing the well-being of your kidneys.

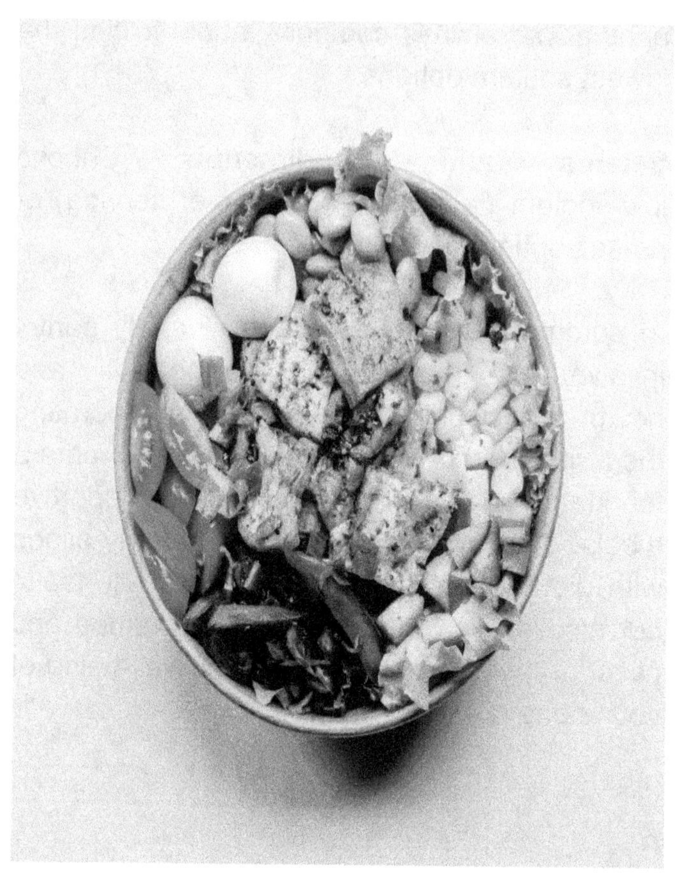

CHAPTER THREE

DELICIOUS AND KIDNEY-FRIENDLY BREAKFAST RECIPES

Berry Blast Overnight Oats

Preparation Time: 10 minutes
Yield: 2 servings
Calorie Count: 250 calories per serving
Nutritional Information per Serving:
- Low in sodium, phosphorus, and potassium
- Rich in antioxidants, fiber, and essential vitamins

Ingredients:
- 1 cup rolled oats
- 1 cup unsweetened almond milk
- 1/2 cup mixed berries (blueberries, raspberries, strawberries)
- 1 tablespoon chia seeds
- 1 tablespoon chopped nuts (walnuts or almonds)
- 1 teaspoon maple syrup (optional)

Method of Preparation:
1. In a jar, combine oats, almond milk, chia seeds, and honey (if using). Stir well.
2. Gently fold in the mixed berries.
3. Seal the jar and refrigerate overnight.
4. In the morning, top with chopped nuts for added crunch.

Health Benefits:
- Berries are rich in antioxidants, supporting kidney health.
- Oats provide fiber, aiding in blood sugar control.
- Almond milk adds a creamy texture without excess phosphorus.

Substitutes:
- Replace almond milk with a low-phosphorus milk alternative.
- Use flax seeds instead of chia seeds.

Tips:
- Personalize with your favorite nuts and seeds.
- Adjust sweetness to preference.

Egg White Veggie Scramble

Preparation Time: 15 minutes
Yield: 2 servings
Calorie Count: 180 calories per serving

Nutritional Information per Serving:
- Low in sodium, phosphorus, and potassium
- High in protein and essential vitamins

Ingredients:
- 4 egg whites
- 1/2 cup diced bell peppers (assorted colors)
- 1/4 cup diced tomatoes
- 1/4 cup chopped spinach
- 1 tablespoon olive oil
- Salt and pepper to taste

Method of Preparation:
1. Heat olive oil in a pan.
2. Add bell peppers and sauté until slightly tender.
3. Add tomatoes and spinach, cooking until wilted.
4. Pour in egg whites, season with salt and pepper.
5. Scramble until eggs are cooked through.

Health Benefits:
- Egg whites offer high-quality protein.

- Colorful veggies provide vitamins and antioxidants.
- Olive oil adds healthy monounsaturated fats.

Substitutes:
- Use a low-sodium seasoning instead of salt.
- Substitute spinach with kale or other leafy greens.

Tips:
- Pair with whole-grain toast.
- Experiment with different vegetable combinations.

Greek Yogurt Parfait Delight

Preparation Time: 10 minutes
Yield: 1 serving
Calorie Count: 220 calories per serving

Nutritional Information per Serving:
- Low in sodium, moderate in phosphorus and potassium
- High in protein, calcium, and probiotics

Ingredients:
- 1/2 cup plain Greek yogurt
- 1/4 cup granola (low-phosphorus)
- 1/4 cup mixed berries
- 1 tablespoon honey

- 1 tablespoon sliced almonds

Method of Preparation:
1. In a glass or bowl, layer Greek yogurt.
2. Add a layer of granola.
3. Top with mixed berries.
4. Drizzle honey over the berries.
5. Sprinkle sliced almonds for crunch.

Health Benefits:
- Greek yogurt is a great probiotic for gut health.
- Berries offer antioxidants and natural sweetness.
- Almonds add healthy fats and vitamin E.

Substitutes:
- Opt for a low-phosphorus granola.
- Use a sugar-free alternative to honey.

Tips:
- Experiment with different fruits and nuts.
- Choose unsweetened Greek yogurt for better control of sugar.

Quinoa Breakfast Bowl Bliss

Preparation Time: 20 minutes
Yield: 2 servings
Calorie Count: 280 calories per serving

Nutritional Information per Serving:
- Low in sodium, moderate in phosphorus and potassium
- High in fiber, essential amino acids and protein

Ingredients:
- 1 cup cooked quinoa
- 1/2 cup sliced strawberries
- 1/4 cup diced mango
- 2 tablespoons pumpkin seeds
- 2 tablespoons coconut flakes
- 1 tablespoon agave syrup (optional)

Method of Preparation:
1. Divide cooked quinoa between two bowls.
2. Top with sliced strawberries and diced mango.
3. Sprinkle pumpkin seeds and coconut flakes.
4. Drizzle with agave syrup if desired.

Health Benefits:
- Quinoa provides a complete protein source.
- Strawberries and mango offer vitamins and antioxidants.
- Pumpkin seeds add healthy fats and magnesium.

Substitutes:
- Replace agave syrup with a sugar-free sweetener.
- Use chia seeds instead of pumpkin seeds.

Tips:
- Add a dollop of low-fat Greek yogurt for extra creaminess.
- Adjust sweetness based on personal preference.

Sweet Potato Pancakes Extravaganza

Preparation Time: 30 minutes
Yield: 2 servings (4-5 small pancakes)
Calorie Count: 220 calories per serving

Nutritional Information per Serving:
- Low in sodium, phosphorus, and potassium
- High in fiber, beta-carotene, and vitamin C

Ingredients:
- 1 cup grated sweet potato
- 2 eggs
- 2 tablespoons whole wheat flour
- 1/2 teaspoon baking powder
- 1/2 teaspoon cinnamon
- 1/4 cup unsweetened applesauce
- 1 tablespoon olive oil

Method of Preparation:
1. In a bowl, combine grated sweet potato, eggs, flour, baking powder, and cinnamon.
2. Stir in applesauce to bind the mixture.
3. Heat olive oil in a pan over medium heat.
4. Spoon small amounts of the batter into the pan to form pancakes.
5. Cook until golden both sides are golden brown in color

Health Benefits:
- Sweet potatoes are abundant in fiber and antioxidants.
- Whole wheat flour adds fiber and nutrients.
- Cinnamon aids in regulating blood sugar levels.

Substitutes:
- Use almond flour for a gluten-free option.
- Substitute applesauce with mashed banana.

Tips:
- Use a dollop of Greek yogurt as toppings.
- Sprinkle with chopped nuts for extra crunch.

Avocado Toast Fiesta

Preparation Time: 15 minutes
Yield: 2 servings
Calorie Count: 240 calories per serving

Nutritional Information per Serving:
- Low in sodium, moderate in phosphorus and potassium
- High in healthy fats, fiber, and vitamins

Ingredients:
- 2 slices whole-grain bread
- 1 ripe avocado
- 1 tablespoon lime juice
- 1/4 teaspoon chili flakes
- Salt and pepper to taste

Method of Preparation:
1. Toast the whole-grain bread slices.
2. Mash the ripe avocado and spread it evenly on the toast.
3. Drizzle lime juice over the avocado.
4. Sprinkle chili flakes, salt, and pepper to taste.

Health Benefits:
- Avocado provides heart-healthy monounsaturated fats.
- Whole-grain bread adds fiber and nutrients.
- Lime juice adds a burst of flavor without sodium.

Substitutes:
- Use low-sodium whole-grain bread.
- Substitute lime with lemon juice.

Tips:
- For added protein, top with a poached egg
- Garnish with fresh herbs like cilantro or parsley.

Chia Seed Pudding Paradise

Preparation Time: 10 minutes (plus overnight soaking)
Yield: 2 servings
Calorie Count: 200 calories per serving

Nutritional Information per Serving:
- Low in sodium, phosphorus, and potassium
- High in fiber, omega-3 fatty acids, and antioxidants

Ingredients:
- 1/4 cup chia seeds
- 1 cup unsweetened almond milk
- 1/2 teaspoon vanilla extract
- 1 tablespoon maple syrup
- Fresh berries for topping

Method of Preparation:
1. In a bowl, mix chia seeds, almond milk, vanilla extract, and maple syrup.
2. Refrigerate overnight or for at least 4 hours until a pudding-like consistency is achieved.
3. Stir well before serving and top with fresh berries.

Health Benefits:
- Chia seeds are rich in omega-3 fatty acids and fiber.
- Almond milk is a low-phosphorus dairy alternative.
- Berries add antioxidants and natural sweetness.

Substitutes:
- Use a low-calorie sweetener instead of maple syrup.
- Experiment with different plant-based milk alternatives.

Tips:
- Customize with nuts or seeds for added crunch.
- Layer with sliced bananas or kiwi for variety.

Spinach and Feta Omelette Fiesta

Preparation Time: 20 minutes
Yield: 1 serving
Calorie **Count:** 230 calories per serving

Nutritional Information per Serving:
- Low in sodium, phosphorus, and potassium
- High in protein, iron, and vitamins

Ingredients:
- 2 eggs
- 1/2 cup fresh spinach, chopped
- 2 tablespoons crumbled feta cheese
- 1/4 cup diced tomatoes
- 1 tablespoon olive oil
- Salt and pepper to taste

Method of Preparation:
1. In a bowl, beat the eggs and season with salt and pepper.
2. Heat olive oil in a pan over medium heat.
3. Add chopped spinach and cook until wilted.
4. Pour beaten eggs over the spinach.
5. Sprinkle feta cheese and diced tomatoes.
6. Cook until the eggs are set, then fold the omelet in half.

Health Benefits:
- Spinach has a high abundance of vitamins and iron
- Eggs provide high-quality protein.
- Feta cheese adds a burst of flavor without excessive sodium.

Substitutes:
- Opt for low-fat feta cheese.
-You can use kale or Swiss chard in place of spinach

Tips:
- Top with fresh herbs like parsley or dill.
- Serve with a side of sliced cucumber for added freshness.

Spinach and Mushroom Omelette Roll

Preparation Time: 20 minutes
Yield: **2 servings**
Calorie Count: 180 calories per serving

Nutritional Information per Serving:
- Low in sodium, moderate in phosphorus and potassium
- High in protein, vitamins, and minerals

Ingredients:
- 4 large eggs
- 1 cup fresh spinach, chopped
- 1/2 cup mushrooms, sliced
- 1/4 cup feta cheese, crumbled
- 1 tablespoon olive oil
- Salt and pepper to taste

Method of Preparation:
1. In a bowl, empty the eggs and season with salt and pepper to taste then whisk.
2. Heat olive oil in a non-stick pan or skillet.
3. Add chopped spinach and mushrooms, sauté until tender.
4. Pour whisked eggs over the veggies, creating a thin layer.
5. Sprinkle crumbled feta cheese and roll the omelet.

Health Benefits:
- Eggs provide high-quality protein.
- Spinach has a high abundance of vitamins and iron
- Olive oil adds healthy monounsaturated fats.

Substitutes:
- Use egg whites for a lower cholesterol option.
- Replace feta with a low-phosphorus cheese.

Tips:
- Experiment with different veggies for variety.
- Garnish with herbs for added freshness.

Sweet Potato Breakfast Hash

Preparation Time: 30 minutes
Yield: 2 servings
Calorie **Count**: 230 calories per serving

Nutritional Information per Serving:
- Low in sodium, moderate in phosphorus and potassium
- High in fiber, vitamins, and antioxidants

Ingredients:
- 1 medium sized sweet potato (peeled and diced)
- 1/2 cup diced bell peppers (assorted colors)
- 1/4 cup diced onions
- 1 tablespoon olive oil
- 1/2 teaspoon smoked paprika
- Salt and pepper to taste

Method of Preparation:
1. In a non-stick skillet or pan, heat olive oil over medium heat.
2. Add diced sweet potatoes, bell peppers, and onions.

3. Season with smoked paprika, salt, and pepper.
4. Cook until sweet potatoes are tender and slightly crispy.

Health Benefits:
- Sweet potatoes have an abundance of fiber and antioxidants.
- Bell peppers are laced with vitamins A and C.
- Olive oil adds heart-healthy monounsaturated fats.

Substitutes:
- Use a low-sodium seasoning blend.
- Substitute sweet potatoes with butternut squash.

Tips:
- Serve with a poached egg for added protein.
- Experiment with different herbs for varied flavors.

Chia Seed Pudding Parfait

Preparation Time: 15 minutes (plus chilling time)
Yield: 2 servings
Calorie Count: 260 calories per serving

Nutritional Information per Serving:
- Low in sodium, moderate in phosphorus and potassium
- High in fiber, omega-3 fatty acids, and antioxidants

Ingredients:
- 1/4 cup chia seeds
- 1 cup unsweetened almond milk
- 1/2 teaspoon vanilla extract
- 1/2 cup diced mango
- 1/4 cup granola (low-phosphorus)
- 1 tablespoon honey (optional)

Method of Preparation:
1. In a bowl, mix chia seeds, almond milk, and vanilla extract.
2. Refrigerate for at least 2 hours or overnight until a pudding-like consistency forms.
3. In serving glasses, layer chia pudding, diced mango, and granola.
4. Drizzle with honey if desired.

Health Benefits:
- Chia seeds are high in omega-3 fatty acids and fiber.
- Almond milk provides a low-phosphorus alternative to dairy.
- Mango contributes vitamins A and C.

Substitutes:
- Use a sugar-free sweetener instead of honey.
- Experiment with different fruits for variety.

Tips:
- Prepare the chia pudding in advance for a quick morning meal.
- Adjust sweetness and texture by varying the amount of honey and almond milk.

Avocado and Tomato Breakfast Toast

Preparation Time: 15 minutes
Yield: 2 servings
Calorie Count: 220 calories per serving

Nutritional Information per Serving:
- Low in sodium, moderate in phosphorus and potassium
- High in healthy fats, fiber, and vitamins

Ingredients:
- 2 slices whole-grain bread (low-sodium)
- 1 ripe avocado, mashed
- 1 medium tomato, sliced
- 1 tablespoon chopped fresh basil
- Salt and pepper to taste

Method of Preparation:
1. Toast the whole-grain bread slices.
2. Spread mashed avocado evenly on each slice.
3. Arrange tomato slices on top.
4. Sprinkle with chopped basil, salt, and pepper.

Health Benefits:
- Avocado provides heart-healthy monounsaturated fats.
- Whole-grain bread offers fiber and B vitamins.
- Tomatoes contribute vitamins A and C.

Substitutes:
- Use a low-sodium bread option.
- Substitute basil with parsley or cilantro.

Tips:
- Add a dash of lemon juice to the avocado for extra flavor.
- For a balanced meal, serve with a side of fresh fruit.

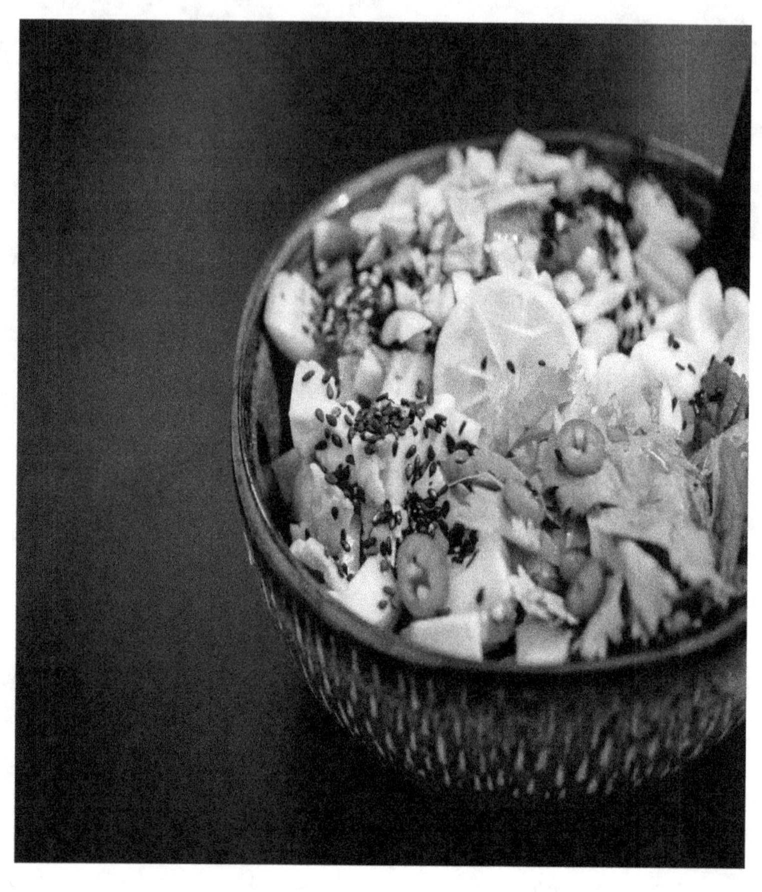

CHAPTER FOUR

SATISFYING LUNCH AND NUTRITIOUS RECIPES

Mediterranean Chickpea Salad Bowl

Preparation Time: 15 minutes
Yield: 4 servings
Calorie Count: 280 calories per serving

Nutritional Information per Serving:
Low in sodium, phosphorus, and potassium
High in fiber, plant-based protein, and essential vitamins

Ingredients:
2 cans (15 oz each) low-sodium chickpeas, drained and rinsed
1 cup cherry tomatoes, halved
1 cucumber, diced
1/2 red onion, finely chopped
1/2 cup Kalamata olives, sliced
1/2 cup crumbled feta cheese

3 tablespoons olive oil
2 tablespoons red wine vinegar
1 teaspoon dried oregano
Salt and pepper to taste

Method of Preparation:
In a large bowl, combine chickpeas, tomatoes, cucumber, red onion, olives, and feta.
In a small bowl, whisk olive oil, red wine vinegar, oregano, salt, and pepper together and set aside
Gently Toss the salad together with the dressing poured on it to combine.
Serve immediately or refrigerate for later.

Health Benefits:
Chickpeas provide plant-based protein and fiber.
Olive oil offers heart-healthy monounsaturated fats.
Tomatoes and cucumbers are rich in vitamins and antioxidants.

Substitutes:
Use low-fat or fat-free feta cheese.
Replace red wine vinegar with balsamic vinegar.

Tips:
Add grilled chicken for extra protein.
Make a big batch and store in the fridge for easy lunches.

Salmon and Quinoa Stuffed Bell Peppers

Preparation Time: 30 minutes
Yield: 3 servings
Calorie Count: 320 calories per serving

Nutritional Information per Serving:
Low in sodium, moderate in phosphorus and potassium
High in omega-3 fatty acids, protein, and fiber

Ingredients:
3 bell peppers, halved and seeds removed
1 cup cooked quinoa
1 can (6 oz) wild-caught salmon, drained
1/2 cup cherry tomatoes, diced
1/4 cup red onion, finely chopped
1/4 cup feta cheese, crumbled
1 tablespoon olive oil
1 teaspoon lemon juice
1 teaspoon dried dill
Salt and pepper to taste

Method of Preparation:
Preheat the oven to 375°F (190°C).
In a bowl, mix quinoa, salmon, tomatoes, red onion, feta, olive oil, lemon juice, dill, salt, and pepper.
Stuff each bell pepper half with the quinoa mixture.
Bake for over 20-25 minutes or until the peppers are tender.

Health Benefits:
Salmon provides omega-3 fatty acids for heart and kidney health.
Quinoa offers fiber and protein.
Bell peppers are laced in vitamins A and C.

Substitutes:
Use canned tuna instead of salmon.
Substitute quinoa with brown rice.
Tips:
For added creaminess, Top with a dollop of Greek yogurt.
Make extra filling for a quick lunch the next day.

Vegetarian Lentil Soup

Preparation Time: 45 minutes
Yield: 6 servings
Calorie Count: 200 calories per serving

Nutritional Information per Serving:
Low in sodium, phosphorus, and potassium
High in plant-based essential minerals protein,
and fiber

Ingredients:
1 cup dry green lentils, rinsed
1 onion, diced
2 carrots, peeled and diced
2 celery stalks, diced
3 cloves garlic, minced
1 can (14 oz) diced tomatoes
6 cups low-sodium vegetable broth
1 teaspoon ground cumin
1 teaspoon ground coriander
1/2 teaspoon smoked paprika
Salt and pepper to taste
2 tablespoons olive oil
Fresh parsley for garnish

Method of Preparation:
In a large non-stick skillet or pot, heat olive oil
over medium heat.
Add onions, carrots, celery, and garlic. Sauté
until vegetables are tender.
Stir in lentils, diced tomatoes, vegetable broth,
cumin, coriander, smoked paprika, salt, and
pepper.

Simmer for 30-35 minutes until lentils are cooked.

Garnish with fresh parsley before serving.

Health Benefits:

Lentils provide plant-based protein and iron.

Vegetables offer vitamins and antioxidants.

Olive oil adds heart-healthy monounsaturated fats.

Substitutes:

Use low-sodium canned lentils for a quicker preparation.

Substitute vegetable broth with low-sodium chicken broth.

Tips:

For a complete meal, serve with a slice of whole-grain bread

Make a large batch and freeze for future lunches.

Citrusy Quinoa Salad with Grilled Chicken

Preparation Time: 30 minutes
Yield: 4 servings
Calorie Count: 310 calories per serving

Nutritional Information per Serving:
- Low in sodium, phosphorus, and potassium

- High in protein, vitamin C and
fiber.

Ingredients:
- 1 cup quinoa, cooked
- 1 pound boneless, skinless chicken breasts
- 1 cup cherry tomatoes, halved
- 1 cucumber, diced
- 1/4 cup red onion, finely chopped
- 2 tablespoons fresh parsley, chopped
- Juice of 2 lemons
- 2 tablespoons olive oil
- Salt and pepper to taste

Method of Preparation:
1. Season chicken breasts with salt and pepper and grill until fully cooked.
2. In a large bowl, combine cooked quinoa, cherry tomatoes, cucumber, red onion, and parsley.
3. Slice grilled chicken and place it on top of the quinoa mixture.
4. In a small bowl, whisk together lemon juice and olive oil. Drizzle over the salad.
5. Toss gently and serve.

Health Benefits:
- Quinoa is laced with essential amino acids and fiber.

- Grilled chicken is a lean source of protein.
- Citrus fruits offer vitamin C for immune support.

Substitutes:
- Use turkey or tofu as a protein alternative.
- Substitute quinoa with brown rice for variety.

Tips:
- Make extra grilled chicken for future meals.
- Add a sprinkle of feta cheese for added flavor.

Zesty Shrimp and Avocado Wrap

Preparation Time: 20 minutes
Yield: 2 servings
Calorie Count: 260 calories per serving

Nutritional Information per Serving:
- Low in sodium, phosphorus, and potassium
- High in omega-3 fatty acids, protein, and healthy fats

Ingredients:
- 1/2 pound shrimp, peeled and deveined
- 1 teaspoon olive oil
- 1 teaspoon chili powder
- 1/2 teaspoon cumin
- 1/4 teaspoon garlic powder
- 2 whole-grain tortillas (low-sodium)

- 1 avocado, sliced
- 1 cup shredded lettuce
- 1/2 cup cherry tomatoes, halved
- 2 tablespoons plain Greek yogurt (optional)

Method of Preparation:
1. In a bowl, toss shrimp with olive oil, chili powder, cumin, and garlic powder.
2. Cook shrimp in a skillet over medium heat until pink and opaque.
3. Warm tortillas in a dry pan or microwave.
4. Assemble wraps with shrimp, avocado, lettuce, and cherry tomatoes.
5. Drizzle with Greek yogurt if desired and fold into wraps.

Health Benefits:
- Shrimp provides omega-3 fatty acids and lean protein.
- Avocados contribute heart-healthy monounsaturated fats.
- Whole-grain tortillas offer fiber for blood sugar control.

Substitutes:
- Make use of chicken or tofu instead of shrimp.
- Choose a low-carb or lettuce wrap for a lighter option.

Tips:
- Personalize with your favorite salsa or hot sauce.
- Add a squeeze of lime for extra zest.

Veggie-Packed Minestrone Soup

Preparation Time: 35 minutes
Yield: 6 servings
Calorie Count: 180 calories per serving

Nutritional Information per Serving:
- Low in sodium, phosphorus, and potassium
- High in fiber, vitamins, and antioxidants

Ingredients:
- 1 tablespoon olive oil
- 1 onion, diced
- 2 carrots, sliced
- 2 celery stalks, diced
- 3 cloves garlic, minced
- 1 zucchini, diced
- 1 can (14 oz) low-sodium diced tomatoes, undrained
- 1 can (15 oz) low-sodium kidney beans, drained and rinsed
- 1 cup green beans, (trimmed and cut into bite-sized pieces)
- 4 cups low-sodium vegetable broth

- 1 teaspoon dried oregano
- 1 teaspoon dried basil
- 1/2 cup whole-grain pasta, uncooked
- Salt and pepper to taste
- Fresh parsley for garnish

Method of Preparation:

1. In a large non stick pot, heat olive oil over medium heat
2. Add onion, carrots, celery, and garlic. Sauté until vegetables are softened.
3. Stir in zucchini, diced tomatoes, kidney beans, green beans, vegetable broth, oregano, and basil.
4. Bring to a boil, and let it simmer on low heat for about 15 minutes.
5. Add pasta and cook until al dente. Season with salt and pepper.
6. Garnish with fresh parsley before serving.

Health Benefits:

- Kidney beans provide plant-based protein and fiber.
- Colorful vegetables offer a variety of vitamins and antioxidants.
- Whole-grain pasta adds complex carbohydrates for sustained energy.

Substitutes:
- Use chickpeas or black beans as an alternative to kidney beans.
- Choose gluten-free pasta for a wheat-free option.

Tips:
- Make a large batch and freeze in individual portions.
- Adjust the pasta amount based on personal preferences.

Feta Stuffed Chicken Breast and Spinach

Preparation Time: 40 minutes
Yield: 2 servings
Calorie Count: 290 calories per serving

Nutritional Information per Serving:
- Low in sodium, phosphorus, and potassium
- High in vitamin K, protein, and iron

Ingredients:
- 2 boneless, skinless chicken breasts
- 2 cups fresh spinach, chopped
- 1/4 cup feta cheese, crumbled
- 1 clove garlic, minced
- 1 tablespoon olive oil

- 1 teaspoon dried oregano
- Salt and pepper to taste
- Lemon wedges for serving

Method of Preparation:
1. Preheat the oven to 375°F (190°C).
2. In a non-stick skillet or pan, heat olive oil over medium heat. Add garlic and sauté until aromatic.
3. Add chopped spinach and cook until wilted. Remove from heat.
4. Cut a slit horizontally into each chicken breast to create a pocket.
5. Stuff each pocket with the sautéed spinach and feta. Season with oregano, salt, and pepper.
6. Bake in the preheated oven for 25-30 minutes or until chicken is cooked through.
7. Serve with lemon wedges for a burst of freshness.

Health Benefits:
- Spinach is abundant in iron and vitamins.
- Feta cheese adds flavor without excess sodium.
- Chicken breast is a lean source of protein.

Substitutes:
- Use goat cheese or a low-sodium cheese alternative.
- Substitute chicken with turkey for a different flavor.

Tips:
- Secure the stuffed chicken with toothpicks before baking.
- Garnish with fresh herbs like parsley or dill.

Turkey and Vegetable Skewers with Quinoa

Preparation Time: 30 minutes
Yield: 4 servings
Calorie Count: 260 calories per serving

Nutritional Information per Serving:
- Low in sodium, phosphorus, and potassium
- Abundant in vitamin A protein, and fiber

Ingredients:
- 1 pound turkey breast, cut into cubes
- 1 zucchini, sliced
- 1 red bell pepper, cut into chunks
- 1 yellow bell pepper, cut into chunks
- 1 red onion, cut into wedges
- 1 cup cherry tomatoes
- 1 cup quinoa, cooked

- 2 tablespoons olive oil
- 1 teaspoon dried thyme
- 1 teaspoon smoked paprika
- Salt and pepper to taste

Method of Preparation:
1. In a bowl, combine turkey cubes, zucchini, bell peppers, red onion, and cherry tomatoes.
2. In a separate bowl, mix olive oil, dried thyme, smoked paprika, salt, and pepper.
3. Marinate turkey and vegetables in the mixture for 15 minutes.
4. Thread turkey and vegetables onto skewers.
5. Grill skewers over medium heat until turkey is fully cooked.
6. Serve over a bed of cooked quinoa.

Health Benefits:
- Turkey is loaded as a lean source of protein
- Colorful vegetables offer vitamins and antioxidants.
- Quinoa is laced with fiber and essential amino acids.

Substitutes:
- Use chicken or tofu as an alternative to turkey.
- Use quinoa with brown rice or couscous as an alternative

Tips:
- Before grilling, soak wooden skewers in water to prevent burning.
- Brush skewers with extra marinade for added flavor.

Lemon Garlic Tilapia with Asparagus

Preparation Time: 25 minutes
Yield: 2 servings
Calorie Count: 240 calories per serving

Nutritional Information per Serving:
- Low in sodium, phosphorus, and potassium
- Abundant in omega-3 fatty acids, protein, and vitamin K

Ingredients:
- 2 tilapia filets
- 1 bunch asparagus, trimmed
- 2 tablespoons olive oil
- 2 cloves garlic, minced
- Juice of 1 lemon
- 1 teaspoon dried thyme
- Salt and pepper to taste

Method of Preparation:
1. Preheat the oven to 400°F (200°C).
2. Place tilapia filets and asparagus on a baking sheet.

3. In a small bowl, mix olive oil, minced garlic, lemon juice, dried thyme, salt, and pepper.
4. Brush the tilapia and asparagus with the lemon garlic mixture.
5. Bake in the preheated oven for 15-18 minutes or until tilapia is flaky and asparagus is tender.

Health Benefits:
- Tilapia is a lean fish rich in protein.
- Asparagus provides fiber, vitamins, and antioxidants.
- Olive oil contributes heart-healthy monounsaturated fats.

Substitutes:
- Use other white fish like cod or sole.
- Substitute asparagus with green beans or broccoli.

Tips:
- Garnish with fresh herbs such as parsley or dill.
- Serve with bed of brown rice or quinoa

Whole Wheat Spaghetti with Fresh Tomato Sauce

Preparation Time: 30 minutes
Yield: 4 servings

Calorie Count: Approximately 300 calories per serving

Nutritional Information per Serving:
- Sodium: Low
- Phosphorus: Low
- Potassium: Low
- Protein: Moderate
- Fiber: High

Ingredients:
- 8 oz whole wheat spaghetti
- 4 large tomatoes, diced
- 2 cloves garlic, minced
- 1/4 cup fresh basil, chopped
- 2 tbsp olive oil
- Salt and pepper to taste

Method of Preparation:
1. Cook the whole wheat spaghetti according to the package instructions.
2. In a separate pan, heat the olive oil and sauté the garlic until fragrant.
3. Add the diced tomatoes and cook until they break down to form a sauce.
4. Season with salt and pepper, then stir in the fresh basil.
5. Toss the cooked spaghetti in the fresh tomato sauce.

6. Serve hot, garnished with additional basil if desired.

Health Benefits:
This dish is rich in fiber, which can help with blood sugar control and promote a feeling of fullness. Whole wheat pasta is a good source of complex carbohydrates, providing sustained energy and being less processed than white pasta.

Substitutes for the Ingredients:
- Whole wheat spaghetti can be substituted with low-potassium pasta options such as rice noodles or shirataki pasta.
- Fresh tomatoes can be replaced with low-sodium, canned diced tomatoes.

Tips:
- To further enhance the flavor, add a sprinkle of grated lemon zest over the pasta before serving.
- Incorporate non-starchy vegetables like sautéed spinach or roasted bell peppers for added nutrition and flavor.

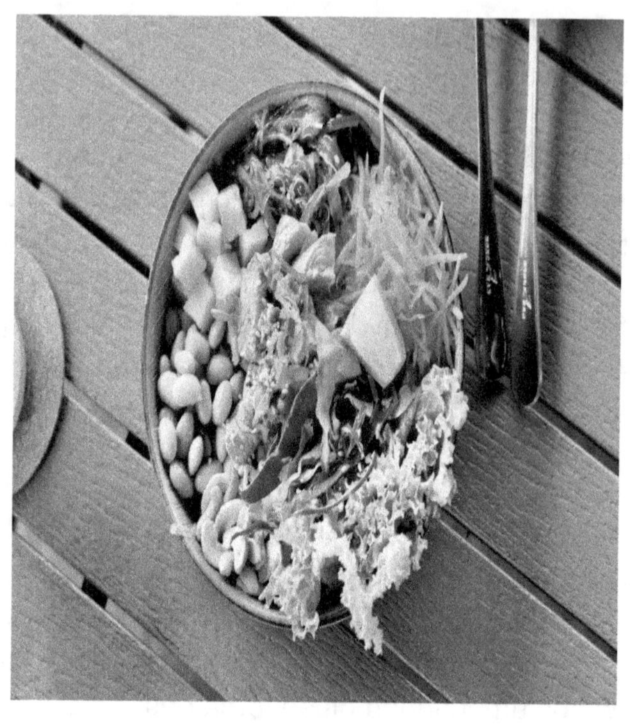

CHAPTER FIVE

DINNER RECIPES

Baked Lemon Herb Salmon with Roasted Vegetables

Preparation Time: 30 minutes
Yield: 2 servings
Calorie **Count:** 300 calories per serving

Nutritional Information per Serving:
- Low in sodium, phosphorus, and potassium
- High in omega-3 fatty acids, lean protein, and antioxidants

Ingredients:
- 2 salmon filets (6 oz each)
- 1 lemon, sliced
- 2 tablespoons olive oil
- 1 teaspoon dried dill
- 1 teaspoon dried thyme
- 1 teaspoon garlic powder

- 2 cups mixed vegetables (zucchini, cherry tomatoes, bell peppers)
- Salt and pepper to taste

Method of Preparation:
1. Preheat the oven to 400°F (200°C).
2. Put the salmon filets on a parchment paper-lined baking sheet
3. Arrange lemon slices on top of the salmon.
4. In a bowl, mix olive oil, dried dill, dried thyme, garlic powder, salt, and pepper.
5. Brush the herb mixture over the salmon.
6. Toss mixed vegetables in the remaining herb mixture and spread around the salmon.
7. Bake for 20-25 minutes or until salmon is cooked through.

Health Benefits:
- Salmon provides omega-3 fatty acids for heart and kidney health.
- Lemon adds vitamin C and a bright flavor.
- Mixed vegetables offer vitamins and fiber.

Substitutes:
- Use trout or tilapia as an alternative to salmon.
- Choose your favorite herbs for the seasoning.

Tips:
- Serve over a bed of quinoa for a complete meal.
- Drizzle with a balsamic glaze for extra depth of flavor.

Spaghetti Squash Primavera with Grilled Chicken

Preparation Time: 45 minutes
Yield: 4 servings
Calorie Count: 250 calories per serving

Nutritional Information per Serving:
- Low in sodium, phosphorus, and potassium
- High in fiber, lean protein, and vitamins

Ingredients:
- 1 medium spaghetti squash
- 2 chicken breasts, grilled and sliced
- 1 cup cherry tomatoes, halved
- 1 zucchini, spiralized
- 1 carrot, julienned
- 2 cloves garlic, minced
- 2 tablespoons olive oil
- 1/4 cup fresh basil, chopped
- Salt and pepper to taste
- Parmesan cheese for garnish (optional)

Method of Preparation:
1. Preheat the oven to 375°F (190°C).
2. Cut the spaghetti squash in half lengthwise, scoop out seeds, and place cut side down on a baking sheet.
3. Bake for 30-35 minutes or until squash is tender.
4. In a skillet, sauté garlic in olive oil until fragrant.
5. Add cherry tomatoes, zucchini, and carrots. Sauté until vegetables are tender.
6. Use a fork to scrape the spaghetti squash into "noodles."
7. Toss the squash noodles with grilled chicken and sautéed vegetables.
8. Garnish with fresh basil and Parmesan cheese if desired.

Health Benefits:
- Spaghetti squash is a low-carb alternative unlike pasta.
- Grilled chicken provides lean protein.
- Vegetables offer vitamins and antioxidants.

Substitutes:
- Opt for shrimp or tofu instead of chicken.
- Substitute spiralized sweet potatoes for added sweetness.

Tips:
- Roast the spaghetti squash in advance for quicker preparation.
- Customize with your favorite veggies and herbs.

Stir-Fried Tofu and Broccoli with Brown Rice

Preparation Time: 35 minutes
Yield: 3 servings
Calorie Count: 280 calories per serving

Nutritional Information per Serving:
- Low in sodium, phosphorus, and potassium
- High in plant-based protein, fiber, and essential nutrients

Ingredients:
- 1 block extra-firm tofu, pressed and cubed
- 2 cups broccoli florets
- 1 bell pepper, sliced
- 1 carrot, julienned
- 2 tablespoons low-sodium soy sauce
- 1 tablespoon sesame oil
- 1 tablespoon rice vinegar
- 1 teaspoon ginger, minced
- 2 cloves garlic, minced
- 2 cups cooked brown rice
- Green onions for garnish

Method of Preparation:
1. In a non-stick wok or large skillet, heat sesame oil over medium-high heat.
2. Add cubed tofu and stir-fry until golden brown on all sides.
3. Push tofu to one side of the wok and add broccoli, bell pepper, carrot, ginger, and garlic.
4. Stir-fry vegetables until crisp-tender.
5. Combine tofu with the vegetables and add soy sauce and rice vinegar.
6. Serve over cooked brown rice and garnish with green onions.

Health Benefits:
- Tofu provides plant-based protein.
- Broccoli offers vitamins A and C.
- Brown rice gives fiber and essential nutrients.

Substitutes:
- Use tempeh instead of tofu.
- Substitute quinoa for brown rice.

Tips:
- Marinate tofu in soy sauce for extra flavor.
- Drizzle with Sriracha for a spicy kick.

Sweet Potato Crust with Mushroom and Spinach Quiche

Preparation Time: 40 minutes
Yield: 6 servings
Calorie Count: 220 calories per serving

Nutritional Information per Serving:
- Low in sodium, phosphorus, and potassium
- High in fiber, vitamins, and antioxidants

Ingredients:
- 2 medium sweet potatoes, peeled and thinly sliced
- 1 cup mushrooms, sliced
- 2 cups fresh spinach, chopped
- 1/2 onion, finely chopped
- 4 large eggs
- 1 cup unsweetened almond milk
- 1/2 cup feta cheese, crumbled
- 1 teaspoon olive oil
- 1/2 teaspoon dried thyme
- Salt and pepper to taste

Method of Preparation:
1. Preheat the oven to 375°F (190°C).
2. Arrange sweet potato slices in a pie dish to form a crust.
3. Bake for 15 minutes or until sweet potatoes are slightly tender.

4. In a skillet, sauté mushrooms, spinach, and onion in olive oil until softened.
5. In a bowl, whisk together eggs, almond milk, dried thyme, salt, and pepper.
6. Pour the egg mixture over the sweet potato crust.
7. Add sautéed vegetables and sprinkle feta cheese on top.
8. Bake for 25-30 minutes or until the quiche is set.

Health Benefits:
- Sweet potatoes provide vitamins A and C.
- Spinach is rich in iron and vitamins.
- Eggs offer high-quality protein.

Substitutes:
- Use a mix of your favorite vegetables.
- Substitute almond milk with regular milk if preferred.

Tips:
- Allow the quiche to cool for a couple of minutes before slicing.
- Customize with your favorite herbs and spices.

Lemon Herb Chicken Skewers with Quinoa Pilaf

Preparation Time: 30 minutes
Yield: 4 servings
Calorie Count: 290 calories per serving

Nutritional Information per Serving:
- Low in sodium, phosphorus, and potassium
- High in lean protein, fiber, and essential amino acids

Ingredients:
- 1 lb. chicken breast, diced into cubes
- 1 lemon, juiced and zested
- 2 tablespoons olive oil
- 1 teaspoon dried rosemary
- 1 teaspoon dried thyme
- 2 cloves garlic, minced
- 1 cup quinoa, rinsed
- 2 cups low-sodium chicken broth
- 1 cup green peas
- 1/4 cup fresh parsley, chopped
- Salt and pepper to taste

Method of Preparation:
1. In a bowl, marinate chicken cubes in lemon juice, lemon zest, olive oil, rosemary, thyme, garlic, salt, and pepper for at least 15 minutes.
2. Thread marinated chicken onto skewers.

3. Grill or broil chicken skewers until fully cooked.

4. In a pot, combine quinoa and chicken broth. Bring to a boil, then reduce heat and simmer until quinoa is cooked.

5. Stir in green peas and fresh parsley.

6. Serve lemon herb chicken skewers over quinoa pilaf.

Health Benefits:

- Chicken breast provides lean protein.
- Quinoa gives fiber and essential amino acids.
- Lemon adds vitamin C and a bright flavor.

Substitutes:

- Use brown rice instead of quinoa.
- Substitute chicken with tofu or shrimp.

Tips:

- Soak wooden skewers in water before grilling.
- Drizzle extra lemon juice before serving for a burst of freshness.

Vegetarian Black Bean Enchiladas

Preparation Time: 35 minutes
Yield: 5 servings
Calorie Count: 260 calories per serving

Nutritional Information per Serving:
- Low in sodium, phosphorus, and potassium
- Abundant in plant-based protein, fiber, and vitamins

Ingredients:
- 1 can (15 oz) low-sodium black beans, drained and rinsed
- 1 cup corn kernels (fresh or frozen)
- 1 bell pepper, diced
- 1/2 red onion, finely chopped
- 1 cup enchilada sauce (low-sodium)
- 10 small whole wheat tortillas
- 1 cup shredded cheese (cheddar or Mexican blend)
- 1 teaspoon cumin
- 1 teaspoon chili powder
- Fresh cilantro for garnish
- Greek yogurt for serving

Method of Preparation:
1. Preheat the oven to 375°F (190°C).
2. In a bowl, mix black beans, corn, bell pepper, red onion, cumin, and chili powder.
3. Warm tortillas and spoon the bean mixture onto each tortilla.
4. Roll up tortillas and place them seam-side down in a baking dish.

5. Pour enchilada sauce over the rolled tortillas and sprinkle with shredded cheese.
6. Bake for 20-25 minutes or until the cheese is melted and bubbly.
7. Garnish with fresh cilantro and serve with a dollop of Greek yogurt.

Health Benefits:
- Black beans provide plant-based protein and fiber.
- Bell peppers offer vitamins A and C.
- Whole wheat tortillas add fiber and complex carbohydrates.

Substitutes:
- Use a dairy-free cheese alternative.
- Opt for gluten-free tortillas if needed.

Tips:
- Customize with your favorite veggies.
- Top with sliced avocado for creaminess.

Balsamic Glazed Salmon with Roasted Vegetables

Preparation Time: 30 minutes
Yield: 2 servings
Calorie Count: 320 calories per serving

Nutritional Information per Serving:
- Low in sodium, phosphorus, and potassium
- Has a high abundance in omega-3 fatty acids, protein, and antioxidants

Ingredients:
- 2 salmon filets (6 oz each)
- 2 cups of mixed vegetables such as cherry tomatoes, bell peppers and zucchini
- 2 tablespoons balsamic glaze
- 1 tablespoon olive oil
- 1 teaspoon dried rosemary
- Salt and pepper to taste
- Lemon wedges for serving

Method of Preparation:
1. Preheat the oven to 400°F (200°C).
2. Place salmon filets and mixed vegetables on a baking sheet.
3. Drizzle with olive oil, balsamic glaze, and sprinkle with dried rosemary, salt, and pepper.
4. Roast for 20-25 minutes or until salmon is cooked through.
5. Serve with lemon wedges.

Health Benefits:
- Salmon provides omega-3 fatty acids for heart and kidney health.
- Mixed vegetables offer vitamins and fiber.

- Balsamic glaze adds flavor without excess sodium.

Substitutes:
- Use other lean fish like cod or tilapia.
- Substitute balsamic glaze with a homemade vinaigrette.

Tips:
- Customize with your favorite veggies.
- Garnish with fresh herbs for extra freshness.

Quinoa and Vegetable Stir-Fry with Tofu

Preparation Time: 35 minutes
Yield: 4 servings
Calorie Count: 280 calories per serving

Nutritional Information per Serving:
- Low in sodium, phosphorus, and potassium
- High in plant-based protein, fiber, and essential nutrients

Ingredients:
- 1 cup quinoa, rinsed
- 1 block extra-firm tofu, cubed
- 2 cups broccoli florets
- 1 red bell pepper, sliced
- 1 carrot, julienned

- 3 tablespoons low-sodium soy sauce
- 1 tablespoon sesame oil
- 1 tablespoon rice vinegar
- 1 teaspoon fresh ginger, minced
- 1 teaspoon garlic, minced
- 1 tablespoon green onions, chopped

Method of Preparation:
1. Cook quinoa according to package instructions.
2. In a large skillet, sauté tofu cubes until golden brown.
3. Add broccoli, bell pepper, and carrot. Stir-fry until veggies are tender-crisp.
4. In a small bowl, whisk together soy sauce, sesame oil, rice vinegar, ginger, and garlic.
5. Add cooked quinoa and sauce to the skillet, toss until well combined.
6. Garnish with green onions before serving.

Health Benefits:
- Tofu provides plant-based protein.
- Quinoa gives fiber and essential amino acids.
- Vegetables add vitamins and antioxidants.

Substitutes:
- Use tempeh as an alternative to tofu.
- Choose tamari for a gluten-free soy sauce.

Tips:
- Marinate tofu in advance for extra flavor.
- Add a dash of sriracha for a spicy kick.

Mushroom and Spinach Stuffed Chicken Breast

Preparation Time: 40 minutes
Yield: 2 servings
Calorie Count: 290 calories per serving

Nutritional Information per Serving:
- Low in sodium, phosphorus, and potassium
- Has a high abundance in lean protein, vitamins, and antioxidants

Ingredients:
- 2 boneless, skinless chicken breasts
- 1 cup mushrooms, chopped
- 2 cups fresh spinach, chopped
- 1/4 cup Parmesan cheese, grated
- 2 cloves garlic, minced
- 1 tablespoon olive oil
- 1 teaspoon dried thyme
- Salt and pepper to taste
- Toothpicks for securing

Method of Preparation:
1. Preheat the oven to 375°F (190°C).
2. In a skillet, sauté mushrooms and garlic in olive oil until softened.
3. Add chopped spinach and cook until wilted.
4. Butterfly each chicken breast and stuff with the mushroom and spinach mixture.
5. Sprinkle with Parmesan cheese, dried thyme, salt, and pepper.
6. Secure stuffed chicken with toothpicks and bake for 25-30 minutes.

Health Benefits:
- Chicken breast provides lean protein.
- Mushrooms offer vitamins and antioxidants.
- Spinach adds iron and essential nutrients.

Substitutes:
- Use feta cheese instead of Parmesan.
- Substitute dried thyme with rosemary.

Tips:
- Serve with a side of roasted sweet potatoes.
- Drizzle with balsamic reduction for extra flavor.

Cauliflower and Chickpea Curry

Preparation Time: 30 minutes
Yield: 4 servings
Calorie Count: 250 calories per serving

Nutritional Information per Serving:
- Low in sodium, phosphorus, and potassium
- High in plant-based protein, fiber, and anti-inflammatory spices

Ingredients:
- 1 head cauliflower, cut into florets
- 1 can (15 oz) of drained and rinsed chickpeas
- 1 onion, diced
- 2 tomatoes, chopped
- 1 can (14 oz) coconut milk
- 2 tablespoons curry powder
- 1 teaspoon turmeric
- 1 teaspoon cumin
- 1 teaspoon coriander
- 1 tablespoon olive oil
- Fresh cilantro for garnish
- Brown rice for serving

Method of Preparation:
1. In a large pot, sauté diced onion in olive oil until translucent.
2. Add curry powder, turmeric, cumin, and coriander. Stir to coat the onions.

3. Add cauliflower florets, chickpeas, and chopped tomatoes. Cook for 5 minutes.

4. Pour in coconut milk, bring to a simmer, and cook until cauliflower is tender.

5. Serve over brown rice, garnish with fresh cilantro.

Health Benefits:
- Cauliflower provides vitamins and fiber.
- Chickpeas offer plant-based protein.
- Turmeric and cumin have anti-inflammatory properties.

Substitutes:
- Use light coconut milk for a lower-calorie option.
- Substitute brown rice with quinoa.

Tips:
- Add a squeeze of lime juice for brightness.
- Customize spice levels to taste.

Shrimp and Avocado Salad

Preparation Time: 20 minutes
Yield: 2 servings
Calorie Count: 300 calories per serving

Nutritional Information per Serving:

- Low in sodium, phosphorus, and potassium
- High in omega-3 fatty acids, lean protein, and vitamins

Ingredients:
- 1 pound shrimp, peeled and deveined
- 2 avocados, diced
- 1 cup cherry tomatoes, halved
- 1/4 cup red onion, finely chopped
- 2 tablespoons lime juice
- 2 tablespoons cilantro, chopped
- 1 tablespoon olive oil
- Salt and pepper to taste
- Mixed greens for serving

Method of Preparation:
1. In a skillet, cook shrimp until pink and opaque.
2. In a large bowl, combine cooked shrimp, diced avocados, cherry tomatoes, and red onion.
3. In a small bowl, whisk together lime juice, olive oil, salt, and pepper.
4. Pour dressing over the shrimp mixture and toss gently.
5. Serve over a bed of mixed greens.

Health Benefits:
- Shrimp provides a low-fat source of protein.

- Avocado offers heart-healthy monounsaturated fats.
- Cherry tomatoes add vitamins and antioxidants.

Substitutes:
- Use lemon juice as an alternative to lime.
- Substitute shrimp with grilled chicken.

Tips:
- Refrigerate for a refreshing, cold salad.
- Customize with your favorite veggies.

Eggplant and Tomato Whole Wheat Pasta

Preparation Time: 35 minutes
Yield: 4 servings
Calorie Count: 270 calories per serving

Nutritional Information per Serving:
- Low in sodium, phosphorus, and potassium
- High in fiber, vitamins, and antioxidants

Ingredients:
- 8 oz whole wheat pasta
- 1 eggplant, diced
- 2 cups cherry tomatoes, halved
- 3 cloves garlic, minced
- 1/4 cup fresh basil, chopped

- 2 tablespoons olive oil
- 1/4 cup Parmesan cheese, grated
- Salt and pepper to taste

Method of Preparation:

1. Cook the whole wheat pasta according to the instructions on the pack.
2. In a skillet, sauté diced eggplant in olive oil until golden brown.
3. Add minced garlic and cherry tomatoes. Cook until tomatoes are softened.
4. Toss cooked pasta, eggplant mixture, and fresh basil in the skillet.
5. Season with salt, pepper, and sprinkle with Parmesan cheese before serving.

Health Benefits:

- Whole wheat pasta provides fiber and essential nutrients.
- Eggplant offers vitamins and antioxidants.
- Tomatoes add lycopene, known for its potential health benefits.

Substitutes:

- Use gluten-free pasta if needed.
- Substitute Parmesan with nutritional yeast.

Tips:
- Drizzle with balsamic reduction for extra flavor.
- Top with pine nuts for added crunch.

Turkey and Vegetable Lettuce Wraps

Preparation Time: 30 minutes
Yield: 4 servings
Calorie Count: 260 calories per serving

Nutritional Information per Serving:
- Low in sodium, phosphorus, and potassium
- High in lean protein, fiber, and vitamins

Ingredients:
- 1 pound ground turkey
- 1 cup mushrooms, finely chopped
- 1 cup bell peppers (assorted colors), diced
- 1/2 cup carrots, julienned
- 1/4 cup hoisin sauce
- 2 tablespoons low-sodium soy sauce
- 1 tablespoon olive oil
- 1 teaspoon fresh ginger, minced
- 1 teaspoon garlic, minced
- 1 head iceberg lettuce, leaves separated

Method of Preparation:
1. In a skillet, cook ground turkey until browned.

2. Add chopped mushrooms, bell peppers, and julienned carrots. Sauté until the veggies are tender.
3. In a small bowl, whisk together hoisin sauce, soy sauce, ginger, and garlic.
4. Pour the sauce over the turkey and vegetable mixture, stir to coat.
5. Spoon the mixture into iceberg lettuce leaves, creating wraps.

Health Benefits:
- Turkey provides a lean source of protein.
- Mushrooms and bell peppers offer vitamins and antioxidants.
- Lettuce serves as a low-calorie alternative to wraps.

Substitutes:
- Use ground chicken or tofu.
- Substitute hoisin sauce with teriyaki sauce.

Tips:
- Customize with your favorite crunchy veggies.
- Drizzle with sriracha for a spicy kick.

<h1>CHAPTER SIX</h1>

HEARTY VEGETABLES

Roasted Garlic Cauliflower Mash

Preparation Time: 30 minutes
Yield: 4 servings
Calorie Count: 120 calories per serving

Nutritional Information per Serving:
- Low in sodium, phosphorus, and potassium
- High in fiber, vitamins, and antioxidants

Ingredients:
- 1 head cauliflower, cut into florets
- 3 cloves garlic, minced
- 2 tablespoons olive oil
- 1/4 cup low-sodium vegetable broth
- Salt and pepper to taste
- Chives for garnish

Method of Preparation:
1. Preheat the oven to 400°F (200°C).

2. Toss cauliflower florets and minced garlic with olive oil, salt, and pepper.
3. Roast in the oven for about 25-30 minutes or until golden.
4. Blend roasted cauliflower with vegetable broth until smooth.
5. Garnish with chopped chives before serving.

Health Benefits:
- Cauliflower is a low-carb substitute for potatoes.
- Garlic contains allicin, known for its anti-inflammatory properties.
- Olive oil adds heart-healthy monounsaturated fats.

Substitutes:
- Use roasted garlic powder instead of fresh garlic.
- Substitute olive oil with avocado oil.

Tips:
- Customize with your favorite herbs.
- Serve as a side dish or a hearty dip.

Baked Herb-Roasted Brussels Sprouts

Preparation Time: 30 minutes
Yield: 4 servings
Calorie Count: 90 calories per serving

Nutritional Information per Serving:
- Low in sodium, phosphorus, and potassium
- High in fiber, vitamins, and antioxidants

Ingredients:
- 1 pound Brussels sprouts, trimmed and halved
- 2 tablespoons olive oil
- 1 teaspoon dried thyme
- 1 teaspoon dried rosemary
- 1 teaspoon garlic powder
- Salt and pepper to taste
- Lemon wedges for serving

Method of Preparation:
1. Preheat the oven to 400°F (200°C).
2. Toss Brussels sprouts with olive oil, thyme, rosemary, garlic powder, salt, and pepper.
3. Spread on a baking sheet in a single layer.
4. Roast for 20-25 minutes or until golden brown and crispy.
5. Squeeze lemon wedges over the roasted Brussels sprouts before serving.

Health Benefits:
- Brussels sprouts have an abundance of fiber and vitamin C.
- Olive oil provides heart-healthy monounsaturated fats.
- Herbs add flavor without excess sodium.

Substitutes:
- Use fresh herbs instead of dried.
- Substitute olive oil with avocado oil.

Tips:
- Add a dash of balsamic vinegar for extra tang.

Eggplant and Tomato Bake

Preparation Time: 40 minutes
Yield: 4 servings
Calorie Count: 160 calories per serving

Nutritional Information per Serving:
- Low in sodium, phosphorus, and potassium
- High in fiber, vitamins, and antioxidants

Ingredients:
- 1 large eggplant, sliced into rounds
- 2 cups cherry tomatoes, halved
- 1/4 cup fresh basil, chopped
- 2 tablespoons olive oil

- 2 cloves garlic, minced
- 1/4 cup grated Parmesan cheese
- Salt and pepper to taste

Method of Preparation:
1. Preheat the oven to 375°F (190°C).
2. Arrange eggplant slices on a baking sheet.
3. In a bowl, toss cherry tomatoes with olive oil, garlic, salt, and pepper.
4. Place tomato mixture on top of each eggplant slice.
5. Bake for 25-30 minutes or until the eggplant is tender.
6. Sprinkle with fresh basil and Parmesan cheese before serving.

Health Benefits:
- Eggplants are very low in calories and high in fiber.
- Tomatoes provide vitamins and antioxidants.
- Olive oil adds heart-healthy monounsaturated fats.

Substitutes:
- Use whole tomatoes, sliced instead of cherry tomatoes.
- Substitute Parmesan cheese with nutritional yeast.

Tips:
- Serve over whole-grain pasta or quinoa.
- Drizzle with balsamic glaze for extra flavor.

Mushroom and Spinach Stuffed Bell Peppers

Preparation Time: 35 minutes
Yield: 3 servings
Calorie Count: 140 calories per serving

Nutritional Information per Serving:
- Low in sodium, phosphorus, and potassium
- High in fiber, vitamins, and antioxidants

Ingredients:
- 3 bell peppers, halved and seeds removed
- 1 cup mushrooms, finely chopped
- 2 cups spinach, chopped
- 1/2 onion, finely chopped
- 2 cloves garlic, minced
- 1 cup cooked quinoa
- 1 teaspoon dried thyme
- 1 teaspoon smoked paprika
- 1/4 cup feta cheese, crumbled
- Salt and pepper to taste

Method of Preparation:
1. Preheat the oven to 375°F (190°C).

2. In a skillet, sauté mushrooms, spinach, onion, and garlic until vegetables are softened.
3. In a bowl, combine cooked quinoa, sautéed vegetables, thyme, smoked paprika, feta cheese, salt, and pepper.
4. Stuff each bell pepper half with the quinoa mixture.
5. Bake for 20-25 minutes or until peppers are tender.

Health Benefits:
- Mushrooms are low in calories and rich in vitamins.
- Spinach provides iron and antioxidants.
- Quinoa adds protein and essential amino acids.

Substitutes:
- Use brown rice instead of quinoa.
- Opt for a vegan cheese substitute.

Tips:
- Customize with your favorite herbs.
- Drizzle with olive oil before serving.

Stuffed Acorn Squash with Quinoa and Cranberries

Preparation Time: 40 minutes
Yield: 4 servings

Calorie Count: 180 calories per serving

Nutritional Information per Serving:
- Low in sodium, phosphorus, and potassium
- High in fiber, vitamins, and antioxidants

Ingredients:
- 2 acorn squash, halved and seeds removed
- 1 cup cooked quinoa
- 1/4 cup dried cranberries
- 1/4 cup pecans, chopped
- 2 tablespoons maple syrup
- 1 tablespoon olive oil
- 1 teaspoon cinnamon
- Salt and pepper to taste

Method of Preparation:
1. Preheat the oven to 375°F (190°C).
2. Place acorn squash halves on a baking sheet, cut side down.
3. Bake for 20-25 minutes or until squash is slightly tender.
4. In a bowl, combine cooked quinoa, dried cranberries, pecans, maple syrup, olive oil, cinnamon, salt, and pepper.
5. Spoon the quinoa mixture into each acorn squash half.
6. Bake for an additional 15-20 minutes or until squash is fully cooked.

Health Benefits:
- Acorn squash is rich in vitamins A and C.
- Quinoa provides protein and essential amino acids.
- Cranberries offer antioxidants and a touch of sweetness.

Substitutes:
- Make use of walnuts or almonds instead of pecans.
- Substitute dried cranberries with raisins.

Tips:
- Drizzle with extra maple syrup if desired.
- Garnish with fresh parsley for a burst of flavor.

Mediterranean Roasted Vegetable Platter

Preparation Time: 30 minutes
Yield: 4 servings
Calorie Count: 180 calories per serving

Nutritional Information per Serving:
- Low in sodium, phosphorus, and potassium
- Has a high abundance of fiber, antioxidants, and essential vitamins

Ingredients:
- 2 zucchinis, sliced
- 1 eggplant, diced
- 1 red bell pepper, sliced
- 1 yellow bell pepper, sliced
- 1 cup cherry tomatoes
- 1 red onion, sliced
- 3 tablespoons olive oil
- 2 cloves garlic, minced
- 1 teaspoon dried oregano
- Salt and pepper to taste

Method of Preparation:
1. Preheat the oven to 400°F (200°C).
2. In a large bowl, toss zucchinis, eggplant, bell peppers, cherry tomatoes, and red onion with olive oil, minced garlic, dried oregano, salt, and pepper.
3. Spread the vegetables on a baking sheet in a single layer.
4. Roast for 20-25 minutes or until vegetables are tender and slightly golden.

Health Benefits:
- Zucchini and eggplant provide fiber and vitamins.
- Bell peppers give antioxidants and vitamin C.
- Olive oil adds heart-healthy monounsaturated fats.

Substitutes:
- Use balsamic vinegar for added flavor.
- Swap cherry tomatoes with grape tomatoes.

Tips:
- Serve over quinoa or whole-grain couscous.
- Drizzle with a lemon-tahini dressing for extra zest.

Balsamic Glazed Brussels Sprouts with Almonds

Preparation Time: 25 minutes
Yield: 4 servings
Calorie Count: 120 calories per serving

Nutritional Information per Serving:
- Low in sodium, phosphorus, and potassium
- High in fiber, vitamin K, and healthy fats

Ingredients:
- 1 pound Brussels sprouts, trimmed and halved
- 2 tablespoons olive oil
- 2 tablespoons balsamic glaze
- 1/4 cup sliced almonds, toasted
- Salt and pepper to taste

Method of Preparation:
1. Preheat the oven to 400°F (200°C).
2. Toss Brussels sprouts with olive oil, balsamic glaze, salt, and pepper in a bowl.
3. Spread on a baking sheet in a single layer.
4. Roast for 20 minutes or until Brussels sprouts are caramelized and crispy.
5. Sprinkle it with toasted sliced almonds before serving.

Health Benefits:
- Brussels sprouts are abundant in fiber and vitamin K.
- Olive oil provides heart-healthy monounsaturated fats.
- Almonds add healthy fats and crunch.

Substitutes:
- Use honey as a natural sweetener.
- Substitute balsamic glaze with reduced balsamic vinegar.

Tips:
- Top with grated Parmesan for extra flavor.
- Serve as a tasty side dish or add to salads.

Sesame Ginger Glazed Carrots

Preparation Time: 20 minutes
Yield: 4 servings

Calorie Count: 100 calories per serving

Nutritional Information per Serving:
- Low in sodium, phosphorus, and potassium
- High in fiber, beta-carotene, and antioxidants

Ingredients:
- 1 pound baby carrots
- 2 tablespoons sesame oil
- 1 tablespoon low-sodium soy sauce
- 1 tablespoon rice vinegar
- 1 tablespoon honey
- 1 teaspoon fresh ginger, grated
- 1 tablespoon sesame seeds, toasted
- Fresh cilantro for garnish

Method of Preparation:
1. Steam or boil baby carrots until tender-crisp, about 5-7 minutes.
2. In a bowl, whisk together sesame oil, soy sauce, rice vinegar, honey, and grated ginger.
3. Toss the steamed carrots in the sesame ginger glaze.
4. Sprinkle with toasted sesame seeds and garnish with fresh cilantro.

Health Benefits:
- Carrots are high in beta-carotene.
- Sesame oil provides healthy fats.

- Ginger adds anti-inflammatory properties.

Substitutes:
- Use maple syrup instead of honey.
- Substitute rice vinegar with apple cider vinegar.

Tips:
- Serve as a scrumptious side dish or snack.
- Garnish with chopped green onions for freshness.

Cauliflower and Broccoli Gratin

Preparation Time: 35 minutes
Yield: 6 servings
Calorie Count: 150 calories per serving

Nutritional Information per Serving:
- Low in sodium, phosphorus, and potassium
- Has a high abundance of fiber, vitamins C and K, and antioxidants

Ingredients:
- 1 head cauliflower, cut into florets
- 2 cups broccoli florets
- 1 tablespoon olive oil
- 2 cloves garlic, minced
- 1 cup low-fat milk
- 2 tablespoons whole wheat flour

- 1 cup shredded low-fat cheddar cheese
- 1/4 cup grated Parmesan cheese
- Salt and pepper to taste
- Fresh parsley for garnish

Method of Preparation:
1. Steam cauliflower and broccoli until just tender, about 5-7 minutes.
2. In a saucepan, heat olive oil and sauté minced garlic until fragrant.
3. Whisk in flour, then gradually add milk, stirring continuously until thickened.
4. Stir in shredded cheddar cheese until it is melted.
5. Combine steamed cauliflower and broccoli with the cheese sauce in a baking dish.
6. Top with grated Parmesan and bake at 375°F (190°C) for 20 minutes or until golden and bubbly.
7. Garnish with fresh parsley before serving.

Health Benefits:
- Cauliflower and broccoli are cruciferous vegetables rich in vitamins and antioxidants.
- Low-fat cheddar provides calcium and protein.
- Olive oil adds heart-healthy monounsaturated fats.

Substitutes:
- Use gluten-free flour for a gluten-free option.
- Substitute low-fat Swiss cheese for cheddar.

Tips:
- Serve as a comforting side dish.
- Add a pinch of nutmeg for extra flavor and warmth.

Spaghetti Squash Primavera

Preparation Time: 40 minutes
Yield: 4 servings
Calorie Count: 160 calories per serving

Nutritional Information per Serving:
- Low in sodium, phosphorus, and potassium
- Has a high abundance of fiber, vitamins A and C, and antioxidants

Ingredients:
- 1 medium spaghetti squash, halved and seeds removed
- 2 tablespoons olive oil
- 2 cloves garlic, minced
- 1 cup cherry tomatoes, halved
- 1 zucchini, diced
- 1 yellow squash, diced
- 1 cup baby spinach
- 1/4 cup fresh basil, chopped

- Salt and pepper to taste
- Grated Parmesan cheese for serving

Method of Preparation:
1. Preheat the oven to 400°F (200°C).
2. Brush the cut sides of spaghetti squash with olive oil and season with salt and pepper.
3. Place squash, cut side down, on a baking sheet and roast for 30 minutes or until tender.
4. While the squash is roasting, sauté minced garlic in olive oil until fragrant.
5. Add cherry tomatoes, zucchini, yellow squash, and baby spinach, cooking until vegetables are tender.
6. Scrape the cooked spaghetti squash into strands with a fork and add to the vegetable mixture.
7. Toss with fresh basil, salt, and pepper.
8. Serve with a sprinkle of grated Parmesan cheese.

Health Benefits:
- Spaghetti squash is a low-carb substitute for pasta.
- Vegetables provide fiber, vitamins, and antioxidants.
- Olive oil adds heart-healthy monounsaturated fats.

Substitutes:
- Use vegan Parmesan for a dairy-free option.
- Substitute spinach with kale or arugula.

Tips:
- Customize with your favorite veggies.
- Top with a dollop of ricotta or feta for creaminess.

Quinoa-Stuffed Bell Peppers

Preparation Time: 35 minutes
Yield: 4 servings
Calorie Count: 240 calories per serving

Nutritional Information per Serving:
- Low in sodium, phosphorus, and potassium
- High in fiber, plant-based protein, and essential amino acids

Ingredients:
- 4 bell peppers, halved and deseeded
- 1 cup quinoa, cooked
- 1 can (15 oz) low-sodium black beans, drained and rinsed
- 1 cup corn kernels (fresh or frozen)
- 1 cup cherry tomatoes, diced
- 1/2 red onion, finely chopped
- 1 teaspoon ground cumin
- 1 teaspoon chili powder

- Salt and pepper to taste
- Fresh cilantro for garnish

Method of Preparation:
1. Preheat the oven to 375°F (190°C).
2. In a bowl, mix cooked quinoa, black beans, corn, cherry tomatoes, red onion, cumin, chili powder, salt, and pepper.
3. Stuff each bell pepper half with the quinoa mixture.
4. Place stuffed peppers in a baking dish and bake for 20-25 minutes.
5. Garnish with fresh cilantro before serving.

Health Benefits:
- Quinoa and black beans provide plant-based protein.
- Bell peppers offer vitamins A and C.
- Corn adds fiber and natural sweetness.

Substitutes:
- Use brown rice instead of quinoa.
- Opt for pinto beans or kidney beans.

Tips:
- For a zesty kick, drizzle with lime juice.
- Serve with a side of salsa for extra flavor.

Crispy Baked Eggplant Parmesan

Preparation Time: 45 minutes
Yield: 4 servings
Calorie Count: 220 calories per serving

Nutritional Information per Serving:
- Low in sodium, phosphorus, and potassium
- Has a high abundance in fiber, antioxidants, and healthy fats

Ingredients:
- 1 large eggplant, sliced into rounds
- 2 eggs, beaten
- 1 cup whole wheat breadcrumbs
- 1/2 cup grated Parmesan cheese
- 2 cups marinara sauce (low-sodium)
- 1 cup shredded mozzarella cheese
- Fresh basil for garnish
- Salt and pepper to taste

Method of Preparation:
1. Preheat the oven to 375°F (190°C).
2. Dip eggplant slices into beaten eggs, then coat with a mixture of whole wheat breadcrumbs, grated Parmesan, salt, and pepper.
3. Place coated eggplant slices on a baking sheet lined with parchment paper.
4. Bake for 25-30 minutes or until crispy.

5. In a baking dish, layer marinara sauce, baked eggplant slices, and shredded mozzarella.
6. Repeat the layers, finishing with a layer of mozzarella on top.
7. Bake for an additional 15 minutes or until the cheese is melted and bubbly.
8. Garnish with fresh basil before serving.

Health Benefits:
- Eggplant provides fiber and antioxidants.
- Whole wheat breadcrumbs add whole grains and fiber.
- Tomatoes in marinara sauce offer vitamins and lycopene.

Substitutes:
- For a gluten-free option, use gluten-free breadcrumbs
- Substitute mozzarella with a dairy-free alternative.

Tips:
- Serve over whole wheat pasta or zoodles.
- Make a large batch and freeze for later.

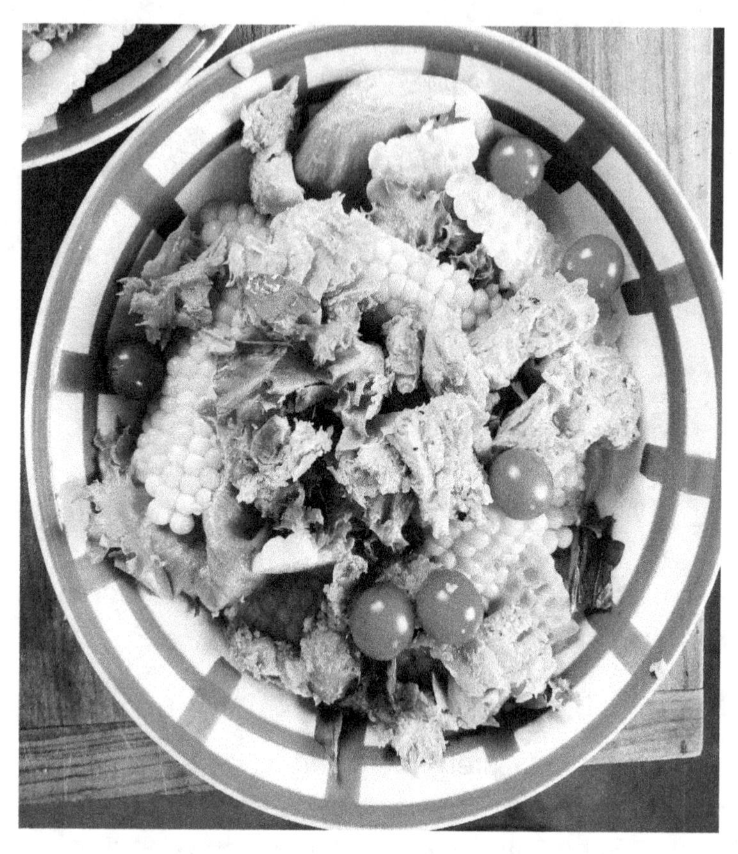

CHAPTER SEVEN

SAVORY SNACKS

Crispy Roasted Chickpeas Trio: Smoky, Spicy, and Herbed

Preparation Time: 35 minutes
Yield: 6 servings (per flavor)
Calorie Count: 120 calories per serving

Nutritional Information per Serving:
- Low in sodium, phosphorus, and potassium
- High in plant-based protein, fiber, and essential minerals

Ingredients for Each Flavor:
For Smoky:
- 2 cans (15 oz each) chickpeas, drained and dried
- 1 tablespoon olive oil
- 1 teaspoon smoked paprika
- 1/2 teaspoon cumin

- Salt to taste

For Spicy:
- 2 cans (15 oz each) chickpeas, drained and dried
- 1 tablespoon olive oil
- 1 teaspoon chili powder
- 1/2 teaspoon cayenne pepper
- Salt to taste

For Herbed:
- 2 cans (15 oz each) chickpeas, drained and dried
- 1 tablespoon olive oil
- 1 teaspoon dried rosemary
- 1 teaspoon dried thyme
- Salt to taste

Method of Preparation:
1. Preheat the oven to 400°F (200°C).
2. In separate bowls, coat chickpeas for each flavor with olive oil and spices.
3. Spread chickpeas in a single layer on a baking sheet.
4. Roast for 25-30 minutes until crispy, shaking the pan occasionally.

Health Benefits:
- Chickpeas are rich in fiber and plant-based protein.
- Smoked paprika and cumin provide antioxidant properties.
- Rosemary and thyme offer anti-inflammatory benefits.

Substitutes:
- Use different spices to suit personal taste.
- Swap chickpeas with black beans for variety.

Tips:
-For a crunchy snack, store in an airtight container.
- Enjoy as a topping for salads or soups.

Zucchini Chips with Herbed Yogurt Dip

Preparation Time: 30 minutes
Yield: 4 servings
Calorie Count: 100 calories per serving

Nutritional Information per Serving:
- Low in sodium, phosphorus, and potassium
- High in fiber, vitamins, and probiotics

Ingredients:
- 2 large zucchinis, sliced into rounds

- 1 tablespoon olive oil
- 1 teaspoon garlic powder
- 1 teaspoon onion powder
- Salt and pepper to taste

For Herbed Yogurt Dip:
- 1 cup Greek yogurt (unsweetened)
- 1 tablespoon fresh dill, chopped
- 1 tablespoon fresh chives, chopped
- 1 tablespoon lemon juice
- Salt and pepper to taste

Method of Preparation:
1. Preheat the oven to 375°F (190°C).
2. Toss zucchini slices with olive oil, garlic powder, onion powder, salt, and pepper.
3. Arrange zucchini on a baking sheet and bake for 20-25 minutes until golden and crisp.
4. Mix Greek yogurt, dill, chives, lemon juice, salt, and pepper for the dip.

Health Benefits:
- Zucchini provides vitamins A and C.
- Olive oil offers heart-healthy monounsaturated fats.
- Greek yogurt gives probiotics for gut health.

Substitutes:
- Use dried herbs if fresh ones are unavailable.

- Substitute zucchini with yellow squash.

Tips:
- Experiment with different herb combinations.
- Dip zucchini chips generously for added flavor.

Cheesy Cauliflower Popcorn Bites

Preparation Time: 40 minutes
Yield: 5 servings
Calorie Count: 150 calories per serving

Nutritional Information per Serving:
- Low in sodium, phosphorus, and potassium
- High in fiber, vitamins, and calcium

Ingredients:
- 1 small cauliflower head, cut into bite-sized florets
- 1 cup whole-grain breadcrumbs
- 1/2 cup Parmesan cheese, grated
- 2 eggs, beaten
- 1 teaspoon garlic powder
- 1 teaspoon onion powder
- Salt and pepper to taste

Method of Preparation:
1. Preheat the oven to 375°F (190°C).

2. Dip cauliflower florets in beaten eggs and coat with a mixture of breadcrumbs, Parmesan, garlic powder, onion powder, salt, and pepper.
3. Place on a baking sheet and bake for 20-25 minutes until golden and crispy.

Health Benefits:
- Cauliflower provides vitamins K and C.
- Whole-grain bread crumbs offer fiber and essential nutrients.
- Parmesan cheese adds calcium for bone health.

Substitutes:
- Use nutritional yeast for a dairy-free alternative.
- Substitute whole-grain breadcrumbs with almond flour.

Tips:
- Serve with a marinara dipping sauce.
- Sprinkle with fresh herbs before baking.

Avocado and Tomato Salsa with Baked Pita Chips

Preparation Time: 25 minutes
Yield: 6 servings
Calorie Count: 130 calories per serving

Nutritional Information per Serving:
- Low in sodium, phosphorus, and potassium
- High in healthy fats, vitamins, and antioxidants

Ingredients:
- 2 avocados, diced
- 1 cup cherry tomatoes, diced
- 1/4 cup red onion, finely chopped
- 1/4 cup fresh cilantro, chopped
- 1 lime, juiced
- Salt and pepper to taste

For Baked Pita Chips:
- 4 whole-grain pita bread rounds, cut into triangles
- 1 tablespoon olive oil
- 1 teaspoon garlic powder
- 1 teaspoon paprika
- Salt to taste

Method of Preparation:
1. In a bowl, combine diced avocados, tomatoes, red onion, cilantro, lime juice, salt, and pepper to make the salsa.
2. Preheat the oven to 375°F (190°C).
3. Toss pita triangles with olive oil, garlic powder, paprika, and salt.

4. Arrange on a baking sheet and bake for 8-10 minutes until crisp.

Health Benefits:
- Avocados provide heart-healthy monounsaturated fats.
- Tomatoes offer vitamins A and C.
- Whole-grain pita adds fiber and complex carbohydrates.

Substitutes:
- Use lemon juice instead of lime.
- Substitute whole-grain pita with gluten-free pita.

Tips:
- Customize salsa with diced jalapeños for heat.
- Serve pita chips warm for the best crunch.

Sweet Potato and Kale Chips

Preparation Time: 30 minutes
Yield: 4 servings
Calorie Count: 110 calories per serving

Nutritional Information per Serving:
- Low in sodium, phosphorus, and potassium
- High in fiber, vitamins, and antioxidants

Ingredients:
- 2 large sweet potatoes, thinly sliced
- 2 cups kale, stems removed and torn into pieces
- 1 tablespoon olive oil
- 1 teaspoon smoked paprika
- Salt and pepper to taste

Method of Preparation:
1. Preheat the oven to 375°F (190°C).
2. Toss sweet potato slices and kale with olive oil, smoked paprika, salt, and pepper.
3. Arrange on baking sheets in a single layer.
4. Bake for 20-25 minutes until crispy.

Health Benefits:
- Sweet potatoes provide vitamins A and C.
- Kale offers vitamins K and A.
- Olive oil adds heart-healthy monounsaturated fats.

Substitutes:
- Use regular potatoes for a different flavor.
- Substitute kale with Swiss chard.

Tips:
- Sprinkle with nutritional yeast for a cheesy flavor.
- Rotate baking sheets for even crisping.

Caprese Skewers with Balsamic Glaze

Preparation Time: 20 minutes
Yield: 6 servings
Calorie Count: 90 calories per serving

Nutritional Information per Serving:
- Low in sodium, phosphorus, and potassium
- Moderate in healthy fats, vitamins, and antioxidants

Ingredients:
- 18 cherry tomatoes
- 18 fresh mozzarella balls
- 18 basil leaves
- 2 tablespoons balsamic glaze

Method of Preparation:
1. Thread cherry tomatoes, mozzarella balls, and basil leaves onto toothpicks or small skewers.
2. Arrange on a serving platter.
3. Drizzle balsamic glaze over the skewers before serving.

Health Benefits:
- Tomatoes offer vitamins A and C.
- Mozzarella provides calcium and protein.

- Basil adds flavor and anti-inflammatory compounds.

Substitutes:
- Use balsamic reduction instead of glaze.
- Substitute mozzarella with a plant-based alternative.

Tips:
- Choose colorful tomatoes for visual appeal.
- Serve as an appetizer for gatherings.

Edamame and Roasted Garlic Hummus

Preparation Time: 25 minutes
Yield: 8 servings
Calorie Count: 100 calories per serving

Nutritional Information per Serving:
- Low in sodium, phosphorus, and potassium
- Highly abundant in plant-based protein, fiber, and healthy fats

Ingredients:
- 1 cup edamame, shelled and cooked
- 1 can (15 oz) of drained and rinsed chickpeas
- 3 tablespoons tahini
- 3 tablespoons olive oil
- 1 head roasted garlic

- 1 lemon, juiced
- Salt and pepper to taste

Method of Preparation:
1. In a food processor, combine edamame, chickpeas, tahini, olive oil, roasted garlic, lemon juice, salt, and pepper.
2. Blend until smooth, adding water if needed for desired consistency.

Health Benefits:
- Edamame and chickpeas offer plant-based protein.
- Tahini provides healthy fats and minerals.
- Roasted garlic adds flavor and anti-inflammatory compounds.

Substitutes:
- Use almond butter instead of tahini.
- Substitute chickpeas with white beans.

Tips:
- Customize with your favorite herbs and spices.
- Serve with whole-grain crackers or sliced veggies

Rosemary and Parmesan Chickpea Crunch

Preparation Time: 25 minutes
Yield: 6 servings
Calorie Count: 120 calories per serving

Nutritional Information per Serving:
- Low in sodium, phosphorus, and potassium
- High in fiber, plant-based protein, and essential amino acids

Ingredients:
- 2 cans (15 oz each) chickpeas, drained and patted dry
- 2 tablespoons olive oil
- 1 tablespoon fresh rosemary, chopped
- 2 tablespoons Parmesan cheese, grated
- 1/2 teaspoon garlic powder
- Salt and pepper to taste

Method of Preparation:
1. Preheat the oven to 400°F (200°C).
2. In a bowl, toss chickpeas with olive oil, rosemary, Parmesan, garlic powder, salt, and pepper.
3. Spread chickpeas on a baking sheet in a single layer.
4. Bake for 20-25 minutes, stirring halfway through, until golden and crispy.

5. Allow to cool before serving.

Health Benefits:
- Chickpeas provide plant-based protein and fiber.
- Olive oil adds heart-healthy monounsaturated fats.
- Rosemary contains antioxidants with potential anti-inflammatory effects.

Substitutes:
- Use nutritional yeast as a dairy-free alternative to Parmesan.
- Substitute rosemary with thyme or oregano.

Tips:
- Store in an airtight container for a grab-and-go snack.
- Experiment with different herbs for flavor variations.

Spicy Edamame Nibbles

Preparation Time: 15 minutes
Yield: 4 servings
Calorie Count: 90 calories per serving

Nutritional Information per Serving:
- Low in sodium, phosphorus, and potassium

- High in plant-based protein, fiber, and essential nutrients

Ingredients:
- 2 cups frozen edamame, thawed
- 1 tablespoon sesame oil
- 1 teaspoon chili powder
- 1/2 teaspoon cayenne pepper
- 1/2 teaspoon garlic powder
- Salt to taste

Method of Preparation:
1. Steam or boil edamame according to package instructions.
2. In a bowl, toss edamame with sesame oil, chili powder, cayenne pepper, garlic powder, and salt.
3. Serve immediately as a zesty, protein-packed snack.

Health Benefits:
- Edamame is rich in plant-based protein and fiber.
- Sesame oil provides heart-healthy unsaturated fats.
- Spices like chili powder and cayenne pepper may boost metabolism.

Substitutes:
- Use olive oil as an alternative to sesame oil.
- Adjust spice levels according to personal preference.

Tips:
- Enjoy with a squeeze of lime for added freshness.
- Sprinkle with sesame seeds for extra crunch.

Baked Sweet Potato Chips

Preparation Time: 30 minutes
Yield: 3 servings
Calorie Count: 110 calories per serving

Nutritional Information per Serving:
- Low in sodium, phosphorus, and potassium
- High in fiber, vitamins, and antioxidants

Ingredients:
- 2 sweet potatoes, thinly sliced
- 2 tablespoons olive oil
- 1 teaspoon paprika
- 1/2 teaspoon garlic powder
- 1/2 teaspoon onion powder
- Salt and pepper to taste

Method of Preparation:
1. Preheat the oven to 400°F (200°C).

2. In a bowl, toss sweet potato slices with olive oil, paprika, garlic powder, onion powder, salt, and pepper.

3. Arrange slices on a baking sheet in a single layer.

4. Bake for about 20-25 minutes, flipping halfway through, until crispy.

Health Benefits:
- Sweet potatoes offer vitamins A and C.
- Olive oil provides heart-healthy monounsaturated fats.
- Baking preserves nutrients compared to deep frying.

Substitutes:
- Use sweet potatoes of different colors for variety.
- Experiment with smoked paprika for a unique flavor.

Tips:
- Allow chips to cool for maximum crispiness.
- Dip in a homemade Greek yogurt-based ranch dressing.

Tomato Basil Bruschetta

Preparation Time: 20 minutes
Yield: 5 servings

Calorie Count: 80 calories per serving

Nutritional Information per Serving:
- Low in sodium, phosphorus, and potassium
- High in vitamins, antioxidants, and heart-healthy fats

Ingredients:
- 3 cups cherry tomatoes, diced
- 1/4 cup fresh basil, chopped
- 2 tablespoons extra-virgin olive oil
- 2 cloves garlic, minced
- 1 tablespoon balsamic vinegar
- Salt and pepper to taste
- Whole-grain baguette slices

Method of Preparation:
1. In a bowl, combine diced tomatoes, chopped basil, minced garlic, olive oil, balsamic vinegar, salt, and pepper.
2. Let the mixture sit for 15 minutes to allow flavors to meld.
3. Toast whole-grain baguette slices until golden.
4. Spoon tomato basil mixture onto each slice and serve.

Health Benefits:
- Tomatoes are rich in vitamins A and C.

- Basil adds a dose of antioxidants.
- Olive oil contributes heart-healthy monounsaturated fats.

Substitutes:
- Use balsamic glaze as a sweeter alternative.
- Opt for gluten-free bread if needed.

Tips:
- Customize with diced red onion for extra crunch.
- Drizzle with a touch of honey for sweetness.

Greek Yogurt and Berry Parfait

Preparation Time: 15 minutes
Yield: 2 servings
Calorie Count: 150 calories per serving

Nutritional Information per Serving:
- Low in sodium, phosphorus, and potassium
- High in protein, calcium, and antioxidants

Ingredients:
- 1 cup Greek yogurt (unsweetened)
- 1/2 cup mixed berries (strawberries, blueberries, raspberries)
- 2 tablespoons honey
- 1/4 cup granola (low-sugar)
- 1/2 teaspoon vanilla extract

Method of Preparation:

1. In a glass or bowl, layer Greek yogurt with mixed berries.
2. Drizzle honey over the berries.
3. Sprinkle granola on top for crunch.
4. Repeat the layers and finish with a dash of vanilla extract.

Health Benefits:

- Greek yogurt is a source of protein and probiotics.
- Berries provide antioxidants and vitamins.
- Honey offers natural sweetness and potential anti-inflammatory properties.

Substitutes:

- Use dairy-free yogurt for a vegan alternative.
- Choose a granola with low added sugars.

Tips:

- Experiment with different fruits for variety.
- Add a sprinkle of chia seeds for extra fiber.

Crunchy Almond-Coconut Energy Bites

Preparation Time: 20 minutes
Yield: 15 bites

Calorie Count: 90 calories per bite

Nutritional Information per Serving:
- Low in sodium, phosphorus, and potassium
- High in protein, fiber, and healthy fats

Ingredients:
- 1 cup rolled oats
- 1/2 cup almond butter (unsweetened)
- 1/4 cup honey
- 1/4 cup shredded coconut (unsweetened)
- 1/4 cup almonds, chopped
- 1/2 teaspoon vanilla extract
- Pinch of salt

Method of Preparation:
1. In a bowl, combine rolled oats, almond butter, honey, shredded coconut, chopped almonds, vanilla extract, and a pinch of salt.
2. Mix until well combined.
3. Refrigerate for 10 minutes to firm up the mixture.
4. With wet hands, roll the mixture into bite-sized balls.
5. Store in the refrigerator until ready to enjoy.

Health Benefits:
- Almonds provide protein and heart-healthy monounsaturated fats.

- Oats offer fiber and sustained energy.
- Honey adds natural sweetness with potential anti-inflammatory properties.

Substitutes:
- Use sunflower butter for a nut-free alternative.
- Opt for maple syrup as a vegan sweetener.

Tips:
- Roll bites in extra shredded coconut for a coating.
- Add a touch of cinnamon for warmth.

Roasted Red Pepper Hummus with Veggie Sticks

Preparation Time: 15 minutes
Yield: 8 servings
Calorie Count: 70 calories per serving

Nutritional Information per Serving:
- Low in sodium, phosphorus, and potassium
- Highly abundant in plant-based protein, fiber, and vitamins

Ingredients:
- 1 can (15 oz) of drained and rinsed chickpeas
- 1/2 cup roasted red peppers, drained
- 1/4 cup tahini

- 2 tablespoons olive oil
- 1 clove garlic, minced
- 1 teaspoon cumin
- Juice of 1 lemon
- Salt and pepper to taste
- Assorted vegetable sticks (carrots, cucumber, bell peppers)

Method of Preparation:
1. In a food processor, blend chickpeas, roasted red peppers, tahini, olive oil, minced garlic, cumin, lemon juice, salt, and pepper until smooth.
2. Adjust seasoning to taste.
3. Serve hummus with assorted vegetable sticks for dipping.

Health Benefits:
- Chickpeas provide plant-based protein and fiber.
- Roasted red peppers offer vitamins A and C.
- Tahini adds healthy fats and a creamy texture.

Substitutes:
- Use almond butter as an alternative to tahini.
- For a smoky flavor, add a pinch of smoked paprika

Tips:
- Make a larger batch and refrigerate for quick snacks.
- Experiment with different veggies for dipping.

Savory Avocado Rice Cakes

Preparation Time: 10 minutes
Yield: 4 servings
Calorie Count: 100 calories per serving

Nutritional Information per Serving:
- Low in sodium, phosphorus, and potassium
- High in heart-healthy fats, fiber, and essential nutrients

Ingredients:
- 4 rice cakes (whole-grain, low-sodium)
- 2 avocados, sliced
- 1 tablespoon lemon juice
- 1 teaspoon chili flakes
- Salt and pepper to taste
- Fresh cilantro for garnish

Method of Preparation:
1. Arrange rice cakes on a serving plate.
2. In a bowl, toss sliced avocados with lemon juice, chili flakes, salt, and pepper.
3. Spoon the avocado mixture onto each rice cake.

4. Garnish with fresh cilantro and serve.

Health Benefits:
-     Avocados provide heart-healthy monounsaturated fats.
- Whole-grain rice cakes offer fiber and sustained energy.
- Lemon juice adds vitamin C for immune support.

Substitutes:
- Use lime juice for a citrusy twist.
- Sprinkle with nutritional yeast for a cheesy flavor.

Tips:
- Top with cherry tomatoes for extra freshness.
- Drizzle with balsamic glaze for added flavor.

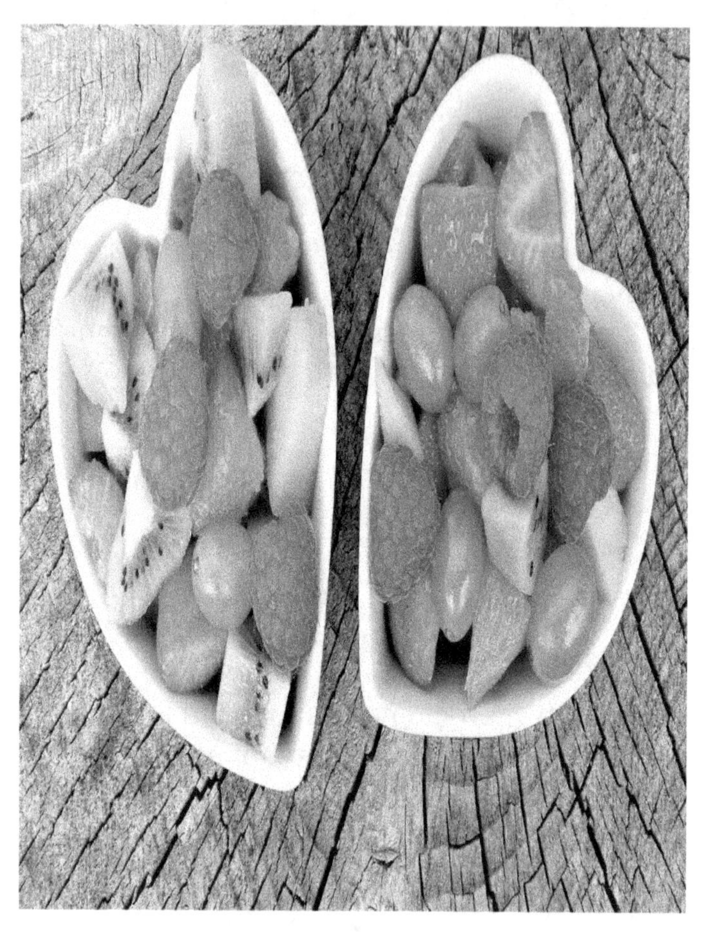

CHAPTER EIGHT

DESERTS AND DRINKS

Cinnamon Baked Apples

Preparation Time: 30 minutes
Yield: 4 servings
Calorie Count: 120 calories per serving

Nutritional Information per Serving:
- Low in sodium, phosphorus, and potassium
- High in fiber, vitamins, and antioxidants

Ingredients:
- 4 apples, cored and halved
- 2 tablespoons melted coconut oil
- 2 tablespoons maple syrup
- 1 teaspoon ground cinnamon
- 1/4 cup chopped walnuts
- Greek yogurt for serving

Method of Preparation:
1. Preheat the oven to 375°F (190°C).
2. Place apple halves in a baking dish.
3. In a bowl, mix melted coconut oil, maple syrup, and ground cinnamon.
4. Brush the mixture over apple halves.
5. Bake for 20-25 minutes or until the apples are tender.
6. Sprinkle chopped walnuts on top.
7. Serve warm with a dollop of Greek yogurt.

Health Benefits:
- Apples provide fiber and vitamins.
- Cinnamon helps regulate blood sugar.
- Walnuts offer omega-3 fatty acids.

Substitutes:
- Use honey instead of maple syrup.
- Substitute walnuts with almonds.

Tips:
- Add a dash of nutmeg for extra flavor and warmth.
-You can also drizzle with a bit of honey before serving.

Coconut Berry Smoothie Bowl

Preparation Time: 10 minutes
Yield: 2 servings

Calorie Count: 160 calories per serving

Nutritional Information per Serving:
- Low in sodium, phosphorus, and potassium
- High in fiber, vitamins, and antioxidants

Ingredients:
- 1 cup mixed berries (strawberries, blueberries, raspberries)
- 1 ripe banana, frozen
- 1/2 cup coconut milk (unsweetened)
- 2 tablespoons chia seeds
- 1/4 cup granola
- Coconut flakes for garnish

Method of Preparation:
1. In a blender, combine mixed berries, frozen banana, coconut milk, and chia seeds.
2. Blend until smooth and creamy.
3. Pour the smoothie into bowls.
4. Top with granola and coconut flakes.

Health Benefits:
- Berries offer antioxidants and vitamins.
- Bananas add natural sweetness and potassium.
- Chia seeds give omega-3 fatty acids and fiber.

Substitutes:
- Use almond milk instead of coconut milk.
- Substitute chia seeds with flax seeds.

Tips:
- Customize with your favorite toppings.
- Drizzle with honey for extra sweetness.

Baked Almond-Orange Ricotta Pancakes

Preparation Time: 25 minutes
Yield: 4 servings
Calorie Count: 220 calories per serving

Nutritional Information per Serving:
- Low in sodium, phosphorus, and potassium
- Has an abundance of protein, vitamins, and healthy fats

Ingredients:
- 1 cup ricotta cheese
- 3 eggs
- 1/4 cup almond flour
- Zest of 1 orange
- 1 tablespoon almond butter
- 1 teaspoon vanilla extract
- 1/2 teaspoon baking powder
- Pinch of salt
- Cooking spray

Method of Preparation:
1. In a bowl, whisk ricotta cheese, eggs, almond flour, orange zest, almond butter, vanilla extract, baking powder, and a pinch of salt.
2. Preheat the oven to 375°F (190°C).
3. Grease a baking dish with cooking spray.
4. Empty the batter into the baking dish.
5. Bake for 20 minutes or until set and golden.

Health Benefits:
- Ricotta cheese is laced with protein and calcium.
- Almond flour adds healthy fats and vitamin E.
- Oranges provide vitamin C and natural sweetness.

Substitutes:
- Use coconut flour for a gluten-free option.
- Substitute almond butter with peanut butter.

Tips:
- Serve with a dollop of Greek yogurt or fresh berries
- Drizzle with a bit of honey for extra flavor.

Minty Watermelon Slush

Preparation Time: 15 minutes

Yield: 2 servings
Calorie Count: 80 calories per serving

Nutritional Information per Serving:
- Low in sodium, phosphorus, and potassium
- Hydrating, rich in vitamins, and antioxidants

Ingredients:
- 4 cups watermelon, cubed and frozen
- 1/4 cup fresh mint leaves
- Juice of 1 lime
- 1 tablespoon honey (optional)
- Ice cubes for serving

Method of Preparation:
1. In a blender, combine frozen watermelon, fresh mint leaves, lime juice, and honey (if using).
2. Blend until smooth.
3. Pour the slush into glasses over ice cubes.

Health Benefits:
- Watermelon is hydrating and loaded with vitamins A and C.
- Mint aids digestion and adds a refreshing flavor.
- Lime juice provides vitamin C.

Substitutes:
- Use agave nectar instead of honey.
- Add a splash of coconut water for extra hydration.

Tips:
- You can garnish with mint leaves for an extra touch.
- Experiment with other frozen fruits for variety.

Cocoa-Dusted Almonds

Preparation Time: 15 minutes
Yield: 8 servings
Calorie Count: 120 calories per serving

Nutritional Information per Serving:
- Low in sodium, phosphorus, and potassium
- Has a high abundance of fiber, healthy fats, and antioxidants

Ingredients:
- 2 cups raw almonds
- 2 tablespoons unsweetened cocoa powder
- 2 tablespoons maple syrup
- 1/2 teaspoon vanilla extract
- Pinch of sea salt

Method of Preparation:
1. Preheat the oven to 325°F (163°C).

2. In a bowl, mix almonds, cocoa powder, maple syrup, vanilla extract, and a pinch of sea salt.
3. Spread out the mixture on a baking sheet lined with parchment paper.
4. Bake for 10-12 minutes, stirring halfway through.

Health Benefits:

- Almonds give healthy fats and vitamin E.
- Cocoa powder is rich in antioxidants.
- Maple syrup adds natural sweetness.

Substitutes:

- Use honey as a substitute to maple syrup and a sprinkle of cinnamon for extra flavor.

Tips:

- Allow the almonds to cool before serving.
- Store in a sealed container for lasting freshness.

Ginger-Turmeric Golden Milk Latte

Preparation Time: 10 minutes
Yield: 2 servings
Calorie Count: 80 calories per serving

Nutritional Information per Serving:
- Low in sodium, phosphorus, and potassium

- High in anti-inflammatory compounds, antioxidants, and essential nutrients

Ingredients:
- 2 cups unsweetened almond milk
- 1 teaspoon ground turmeric
- 1/2 teaspoon ground ginger
- 1 tablespoon honey (optional)
- 1/4 teaspoon ground cinnamon
- 1/4 teaspoon vanilla extract
- Pinch of black pepper (this enhances the absorption of turmeric)

Method of Preparation:
1. In a small saucepan, heat almond milk over medium heat until warm but not boiling.
2. Whisk in turmeric, ginger, honey or maple syrup (if using), cinnamon, vanilla extract, and black pepper.
3. Continue to whisk until well combined and heated through, but do not bring to a boil.
4. Pour into mugs, and enjoy your soothing Ginger-Turmeric Golden Milk Latte.

Health Benefits:
- Turmeric and ginger possess anti-inflammatory properties.
- Almond milk is a dairy-free source of calcium and vitamin D.

- Black pepper enhances the absorption of curcumin which is found in turmeric.

Substitutes:
- Use any plant-based milk (like coconut or oat milk).
- Replace honey with a sweetener of your choice.

Tips:
- Experiment with the sweetness level to suit your preference.
- Sprinkle a dash of nutmeg for added warmth and flavor.

Berry Chia Pudding Parfait

Preparation Time: 30 minutes (+chilling time)
Yield: 4 servings
Calorie Count: 180 calories per serving

Nutritional Information per Serving:
- Low in sodium, phosphorus, and potassium
- High in fiber, antioxidants, and omega-3 fatty acids

Ingredients:
- 1/2 cup chia seeds
- 2 cups unsweetened almond milk
- 1 teaspoon vanilla extract

- 2 tablespoons maple syrup
- 1 cup mixed berries (strawberries, blueberries, raspberries)
- 1/4 cup sliced almonds

Method of Preparation:
1. In a bowl, mix chia seeds, almond milk, vanilla extract, and maple syrup.
2. Refrigerate for at least 4 hours or overnight until the mixture thickens.
3. In serving glasses, layer chia pudding with mixed berries.
4. Repeat layers, finishing with a berry topping.
5. Garnish with sliced almonds before serving.

Health Benefits:
- Chia seeds is loaded with fiber and omega-3 fatty acids
- Berries offer vitamins, antioxidants, and natural sweetness.
- Almonds add healthy fats and a satisfying crunch.

Substitutes:
- Use any plant-based milk that you prefer
- Swap maple syrup with honey for sweetness.

Tips:
- Experiment with different berry combinations and top with a dollop of Greek yogurt for extra protein.

Avocado Chocolate Mousse

Preparation Time: 20 minutes (+chilling time)
Yield: 6 servings
Calorie Count: 150 calories per serving

Nutritional Information per Serving:
- Low in sodium, phosphorus, and potassium
- High in healthy fats, fiber, and antioxidants

Ingredients:
- 2 ripe avocados
- 1/2 cup unsweetened cocoa powder
- 1/4 cup maple syrup
- 1 teaspoon vanilla extract
- Pinch of salt
- Fresh berries for garnish

Method of Preparation:
1. In a blender, combine avocados, cocoa powder, maple syrup, vanilla extract, and a pinch of salt.
2. Blend until smooth and creamy.
3. Refrigerate for at most 2 hours before serving.

4. Spoon into serving bowls and garnish with fresh berries.

Health Benefits:
- Avocados provide healthy monounsaturated fats.
- Cocoa powder offers antioxidants and a rich chocolate flavor.
- Maple syrup adds natural sweetness.

Substitutes:
- Use honey or agave syrup as an alternative sweetener and top with crushed nuts for added texture.

Tips:
- Adjust sweetness to taste.
- Serve with a sprinkle of cocoa nibs for extra crunch.

Greek Yogurt Parfait with Pistachios and Honey

Preparation Time: 15 minutes
Yield: 2 servings
Calorie Count: 200 calories per serving

Nutritional Information per Serving:
- Low in sodium, phosphorus, and potassium
- High in protein, probiotics, and healthy fats

Ingredients:
- 1 cup plain Greek yogurt
- 2 tablespoons honey
- 1/4 cup pistachios, chopped
- 1/2 cup mixed berries (strawberries, blueberries)

Method of Preparation:
1. In serving glasses, layer Greek yogurt with honey, pistachios, and mixed berries.
2. Repeat layers, finishing with a berry and pistachio topping.
3. Drizzle with an extra touch of honey before serving.

Health Benefits:
- Greek yogurt provides probiotics and protein.
- Honey adds natural sweetness and antioxidants.
- Pistachios offer healthy fats and a satisfying crunch.

Substitutes:
- Use any nuts of your choice.
- Substitute honey with maple syrup or agave.

Tips:
- Experiment with different fruit combinations.

- Choose unsweetened Greek yogurt for a lower sugar option.

Coconut Chia Seed Pudding

Preparation Time: 10 minutes (+chilling time)
Yield: 4 servings
Calorie Count: 160 calories per serving

Nutritional Information per Serving:
- Low in sodium, phosphorus, and potassium
- High in fiber, omega-3 fatty acids, and natural sweetness

Ingredients:
- 1 can (13.5 oz) coconut milk
- 1/2 cup chia seeds
- 2 tablespoons maple syrup
- 1 teaspoon vanilla extract
- Shredded coconut for garnish

Method of Preparation:
1. In a bowl, whisk together coconut milk, chia seeds, maple syrup, and vanilla extract.
2. Refrigerate for at least 4 hours or overnight until the mixture thickens.
3. Spoon into serving bowls and garnish with shredded coconut before serving.

Health Benefits:
- Chia seeds offer fiber and omega-3 fatty acids
- Coconut milk offers a creamy texture and healthy fats.
- Maple syrup adds natural sweetness.

Substitutes:
- Use any plant-based milk of your choice and swap maple syrup with honey for sweetness.

Tips:
- Top with fresh berries or sliced mango.
- Layer with granola for added crunch.

Peach and Almond Yogurt Smoothie

Preparation Time: 10 minutes
Yield: 2 servings
Calorie Count: 120 calories per serving

Nutritional Information per Serving:
- Low in sodium, phosphorus, and potassium
- High in protein, vitamins, and antioxidants

Ingredients:
- 2 ripe peaches, pitted and sliced
- 1 cup plain Greek yogurt
- 1/4 cup almond butter
- 1 teaspoon honey

- 1/2 cup ice cubes
- Almond slices for garnish

Method of Preparation:
1. In a blender, combine sliced peaches, Greek yogurt, almond butter, honey, and ice cubes.
2. Blend until smooth and creamy.
3. Pour into glasses and garnish with almond slices before serving.

Health Benefits:
- Peaches offer vitamins A and C.
- Greek yogurt provides probiotics and protein.
- Almond butter gives healthy fats and a nutty flavor.

Substitutes:
- Use any nut butter of your choice and swap honey with maple syrup or agave.

Tips:
- Add a handful of spinach for extra nutrients.
- Customize sweetness by adjusting honey to taste.

Strawberry Banana Oat Smoothie Bowl

Preparation Time: 15 minutes
Yield: 2 servings

Calorie Count: 180 calories per serving

Nutritional Information per Serving:
- Low in sodium, phosphorus, and potassium
- Has a high abundance of fiber, vitamins, and natural sweetness

Ingredients:
- 1 cup frozen strawberries
- 2 ripe bananas
- 1/2 cup rolled oats
- 1 cup unsweetened almond milk
- Toppings: sliced bananas, chia seeds, granola

Method of Preparation:
1. In a blender, combine frozen strawberries, ripe bananas, rolled oats, and almond milk.
2. Blend until smooth and creamy.
3. Pour into bowls and top with sliced bananas, chia seeds, and granola.

Health Benefits:
- Strawberries offer vitamins, antioxidants, and fiber.
- Bananas provide natural sweetness and potassium.
- Oats add fiber for sustained energy.

Substitutes:
- Use any fruit combination of your choice and substitute almond milk with your preferred plant-based milk.

Tips:
- Customize with your favorite toppings.
- Add a spoonful of nut butter for extra creaminess.

Cinnamon Baked Pears with Walnuts

Preparation Time: 25 minutes
Yield: 4 servings
Calorie Count: 140 calories per serving

Nutritional Information per Serving:
- Low in sodium, phosphorus, and potassium
- High in fiber, vitamins, and healthy fats

Ingredients:
- 4 ripe pears, halved and cored
- 1 tablespoon lemon juice
- 1 teaspoon ground cinnamon
- 1/4 cup chopped walnuts
- 1 tablespoon honey

Method of Preparation:
1. Preheat the oven to 375°F (190°C).

2. Place pear halves in a baking dish, cut side up.
3. Drizzle with lemon juice and sprinkle with cinnamon.
4. Top each pear half with chopped walnuts.
5. Bake for 15-20 minutes or until the pears are tender.
6. Drizzle with honey before serving.

Health Benefits:
- Pears provide fiber and vitamins.
- Walnuts offer omega-3 fatty acids and antioxidants.
- Cinnamon adds flavor with potential anti-inflammatory benefits.

Substitutes:
- Use pecans or almonds instead of walnuts.
- Substitute honey with maple syrup or agave.

Tips:
- Serve with a dollop of Greek yogurt.
- Enjoy warm as a comforting dessert.

Matcha Green Tea Smoothie

Preparation Time: 5 minutes
Yield: 2 servings
Calorie Count: 80 calories per serving

Nutritional Information per Serving:
- Low in sodium, phosphorus, and potassium
- High in antioxidants, metabolism-boosting properties, and catechins

Ingredients:
- 1 teaspoon matcha green tea powder
- 1 cup unsweetened almond milk
- 1/2 frozen banana
- 1/2 cup pineapple chunks (fresh or frozen)
- 1/2 cup spinach leaves
- 1 tablespoon chia seeds
- Ice cubes (optional)

Method of Preparation:
1. In a blender, combine matcha powder and almond milk; blend until smooth.
2. Add frozen banana, pineapple chunks, spinach leaves, and chia seeds.
3. Blend until creamy and well combined.
4. If desired, add ice cubes and blend for a colder consistency.
5. Pour into glasses and enjoy immediately.

Health Benefits:
- Matcha green tea is loaded with antioxidants, particularly catechins.
- Spinach provides vitamins A and C, along with iron.

- Chia seeds add omega-3 fatty acids and fiber.

Substitutes:
- Use coconut milk or soy milk instead of almond milk.
- Swap pineapple with mango for a tropical twist.

Tips:
- Adjust sweetness with honey or maple syrup if needed.
- Garnish with a sprinkle of matcha powder for a more visual appeal.

Baked Cinnamon Apple Slices

Preparation Time: 25 minutes
Yield: 4 servings
Calorie Count: 120 calories per serving

Nutritional Information per Serving:
- Low in sodium, phosphorus, and potassium
- High in fiber, vitamins, and antioxidants

Ingredients:
- 4 apples, cored and sliced
- 1 tablespoon lemon juice
- 1 tablespoon honey or maple syrup
- 1 teaspoon ground cinnamon
- 1/4 cup chopped walnuts (optional)

- Greek yogurt for serving

Method of Preparation:
1. Preheat the oven to 375°F (190°C).
2. In a bowl, toss apple slices with lemon juice, honey or maple syrup, and cinnamon.
3. Spread the apple slices on a baking sheet.
4. Bake for 20 minutes or until the apples are tender.
5. Sprinkle with chopped walnuts, if using, before serving.
6. Serve warm with a side of Greek yogurt.

Health Benefits:
- Apples provide fiber and natural sweetness.
- Cinnamon may help regulate blood sugar levels.
- Walnuts offer omega-3 fatty acids.

Substitutes:
- Use a sugar substitute for honey.
- Substitute walnuts with almonds or pecans.

Tips:
- Experiment with different apple varieties.
- Top with a dusting of nutmeg for extra warmth.

Peach and Basil Sorbet

Preparation Time: 15 minutes (plus freezing time)
Yield: 6 servings
Calorie Count: 90 calories per serving

Nutritional Information per Serving:
- Low in sodium, phosphorus, and potassium
- High in vitamins, fiber, and antioxidants

Ingredients:
- 4 ripe peaches, peeled and sliced
- 1/4 cup fresh basil leaves
- 2 tablespoons honey or agave nectar
- 1 tablespoon lemon juice
- 1/2 cup water

Method of Preparation:
1. In a blender, combine peaches, basil, honey or agave nectar, lemon juice, and water.
2. Blend until smooth.
3. Pour the mixture into a shallow dish and freeze for at least 4 hours, stirring every hour.
4. Once fully frozen, scoop the sorbet into serving bowls.

Health Benefits:
- Peaches provide vitamins A and C.

- Basil adds a unique flavor and anti-inflammatory properties.
- Honey or agave nectar sweetens without refined sugars.

Substitutes:
- Use mint instead of basil for a different twist.
- Substitute honey with maple syrup.

Tips:
- Garnish with fresh basil leaves.
- Serve with a slice of fresh peach for presentation.

Coconut Rice Pudding with Mango

Preparation Time: 40 minutes
Yield: 5 servings
Calorie Count: 160 calories per serving

Nutritional Information per Serving:
- Low in sodium, phosphorus, and potassium
- High in fiber, coconut milk benefits, and vitamins

Ingredients:
- 1/2 cup arborio rice
- 1 can (13.5 oz) of light coconut milk
- 1/4 cup honey or maple syrup
- 1 teaspoon vanilla extract

- 1/4 teaspoon ground cinnamon
- 1 ripe mango, diced

Method of Preparation:
1. In a saucepan, combine rice, coconut milk, honey or maple syrup, vanilla extract, and cinnamon.
2. Bring to a boil, then reduce heat and simmer until rice is tender and mixture thickens.
3. Allow the pudding to cool, then refrigerate for at least 2 hours.
4. Serve the pudding topped with diced mango.

Health Benefits:
- Arborio rice provides a creamy texture.
- Coconut milk gives healthy fats and a tropical flavor.
- Mango adds natural sweetness and vitamins.

Substitutes:
- Use brown rice for a whole-grain option.
- Substitute coconut milk with almond milk.

Tips:
- Toast shredded coconut for a crunchy topping.
- Garnish with a sprinkle of ground cardamom.

Lemon Blueberry Yogurt Parfait

Preparation Time: 15 minutes
Yield: 4 servings
Calorie Count: 140 calories per serving

Nutritional Information per Serving:
- Low in sodium, phosphorus, and potassium
- High in protein, vitamins, and antioxidants

Ingredients:
- 2 cups Greek yogurt (unsweetened)
- 1 tablespoon honey or agave nectar
- 1 teaspoon lemon zest
- 1 cup blueberries (fresh or frozen)
- 1/4 cup granola (low-sugar)

Method of Preparation:
1. In a bowl, mix Greek yogurt with honey or agave nectar and lemon zest.
2. In serving glasses, layer the yogurt mixture with blueberries and granola.
3. Repeat the layers, finishing with a sprinkle of granola on top.

Health Benefits:
- Greek yogurt provides protein and probiotics.
- Blueberries offer vitamins and antioxidants.
- Honey or agave nectar sweetens without refined sugars.

Substitutes:
- Use almond or coconut yogurt for a dairy-free option.
- Substitute blueberries with your favorite berries.

Tips:
- Customize with a handful of nuts for crunch.
- Drizzle with a touch of lemon juice for extra zest.

Pumpkin Spice Baked Apples

Preparation Time: 35 minutes
Yield: 6 servings
Calorie Count: 130 calories per serving

Nutritional Information per Serving:
- Low in sodium, phosphorus, and potassium
- High in fiber, vitamins, and antioxidants

Ingredients:
- 6 apples, cored
- 1/2 cup pumpkin puree
- 2 tablespoons maple syrup
- 1 teaspoon pumpkin spice blend
- 1/4 cup chopped pecans
- Greek yogurt for serving

Method of Preparation:
1. Preheat the oven to 375°F (190°C).
2. In a bowl, mix pumpkin puree, maple syrup, pumpkin spice blend, and chopped pecans.
3. Fill each cored apple with the pumpkin mixture.
4. Place the filled apples in a baking dish.
5. Bake for 25-30 minutes or until the apples are tender.
6. Serve warm with a dollop of Greek yogurt.

Health Benefits:
- Apples provide fiber and natural sweetness.
- Pumpkin puree offers vitamins A and C.
- Pecans add healthy fats and a nutty flavor.

Substitutes:
- Use honey instead of maple syrup.
- Swap pecans with almonds or walnuts.

Tips:
- Top with a sprinkle of cinnamon and serve with a scoop of vanilla ice cream if desired.

Mint Chocolate Avocado Popsicles

Preparation Time: 15 minutes (plus freezing time)
Yield: 8 popsicles
Calorie Count: 100 calories per popsicle

Nutritional Information per Serving:
- Low in sodium, phosphorus, and potassium
- High in healthy fats, fiber, and antioxidants

Ingredients:
- 2 ripe avocados
- 1/2 cup cocoa powder (unsweetened)
- 1/4 cup honey or agave nectar
- 1 teaspoon peppermint extract
- 1 1/2 cups almond milk (unsweetened)

Method of Preparation:
1. In a blender, combine avocados, cocoa powder, honey or agave nectar, peppermint extract, and almond milk.
2. Blend until smooth and creamy.
3. Pour the mixture into popsicle molds.
4. Freeze for at least 4 hours or until fully set.
5. Run molds under warm water to release popsicles.

Health Benefits:
- Avocados provide creamy texture and healthy fats.
- Cocoa powder offers antioxidants and a chocolatey flavor.
- Peppermint extract adds a refreshing twist.

Substitutes:
- Use coconut milk instead of almond milk and substitute honey with maple syrup.

Tips:
- Customize with a sprinkle of crushed nuts.
- Experiment with different extract flavors.

Strawberry Basil Lemonade

Preparation Time: 15 minutes
Yield: 4 servings
Calorie Count: 80 calories per serving

Nutritional Information per Serving:
- Low in sodium, phosphorus, and potassium
- High in vitamin C, antioxidants, and hydration

Ingredients:
- 1 cup fresh strawberries, hulled and halved
- 1/4 cup fresh basil leaves
- 1/2 cup freshly squeezed lemon juice
- 2 tablespoons honey or agave syrup
- 4 cups cold water
- Ice cubes
- Lemon slices and basil leaves for garnish

Method of Preparation:
1. In a blender, combine fresh strawberries, basil leaves, lemon juice, and honey or agave syrup.
2. Blend until smooth.
3. Strain the strawberry-basil mixture into a pitcher to remove pulp.
4. Add cold water to the pitcher and stir it well.
5. Fill glasses with ice cubes and pour the strawberry basil lemonade over.
6. Garnish with lemon slices and basil leaves.

Health Benefits:
- Strawberries are rich in vitamin C and antioxidants.
- Basil adds a burst of flavor and potential anti-inflammatory properties.
- Lemon provides refreshing citrus flavor and vitamin C.

Substitutes:
- Use mint leaves instead of basil for a different herbal note.
- Swap honey or agave syrup with stevia for a sugar-free option.

Tips:
- Adjust sweetness to your liking.
-Add sparkling water for a fizzy version

- Make it a frozen treat by blending with ice.

APPENDIX

30 Days Meal Plan

Week 1

Day 1:
- **Breakfast:** Berry Blast Overnight Oats
- **Snack:** Crispy Roasted Chickpeas Trio
- **Lunch:** Mediterranean Chickpea Salad Bowl
- **Dinner:** Baked Lemon Herb Salmon with Roasted Vegetables
- **Dessert:** Cinnamon Baked Apples

Day 2:
- **Breakfast:** Egg White Veggie Scramble
- **Snack:** Zucchini Chips with Herbed Yogurt Dip
- **Lunch:** Salmon and Quinoa Stuffed Bell Peppers
- **Dinner:** Spaghetti Squash Primavera with Grilled Chicken
- **Dessert:** Coconut Berry Smoothie Bowl

Day 3:
- **Breakfast:** Greek Yogurt Parfait Delight
- **Snack:** Cheesy Cauliflower Popcorn Bites
- **Lunch:** Vegetarian Lentil Soup
- **Dinner:** Stir-Fried Tofu and Broccoli with Brown Rice
- **Dessert:** Baked Almond-Orange Ricotta Pancakes

Day 4:
- **Breakfast:** Chia Seed Pudding Parfait
- **Snack:** Avocado and Tomato Salsa with Baked Pita Chips
- **Lunch:** Citrusy Quinoa Salad with Grilled Chicken
- **Dinner:** Sweet Potato Crust with Mushroom and Spinach Quiche
- **Dessert:** Minty Watermelon Slush

Day 5:
- **Breakfast:** Sweet Potato Pancakes Extravaganza
- **Snack:** Sweet Potato and Kale Chips
- **Lunch:** Zesty Shrimp and Avocado Wrap
- **Dinner:** Lemon Herb Chicken Skewers with Quinoa Pilaf
- **Dessert:** Cocoa-Dusted Almonds

Day 6:
- **Breakfast:** Avocado Toast Fiesta
- **Snack:** Caprese Skewers with Balsamic Glaze
- **Lunch:** Veggie-Packed Minestrone Soup
- **Dinner:** Vegetarian Black Bean Enchiladas
- **Dessert**: Ginger-Turmeric Golden Milk Latte

Day 7:
- **Breakfast:** Chia Seed Pudding Paradise
- **Snack:** Edamame and Roasted Garlic Hummus
- **Lunch:** Feta Stuffed Chicken Breast and Spinach
- **Dinner:** Balsamic Glazed Salmon with Roasted Vegetables
- **Dessert:** Avocado Chocolate Mousse

Week 2

Day 8:
- **Breakfast:** Spinach and Feta Omelette Fiesta
- **Snack:** Rosemary and Parmesan Chickpea Crunch
- **Lunch:** Turkey and Vegetable Skewers with Quinoa
- **Dinner:** Quinoa and Vegetable Stir-Fry with Tofu
- **Dessert:** Berry Chia Pudding Parfait

Day 9:
- **Breakfast:** Spinach and Mushroom Omelette Roll
- **Snack:** Spicy Edamame Nibbles
- **Lunch:** Lemon Garlic Tilapia with Asparagus
- **Dinner:** Mushroom and Spinach Stuffed Chicken Breast
- **Dessert:** Greek Yogurt Parfait with Pistachios and Honey

Day 10:
- **Breakfast:** Sweet Potato Breakfast Hash
- **Snack:** Tomato Basil Bruschetta
- **Lunch:** Whole Wheat Spaghetti with Fresh Tomato Sauce
- **Dinner:** Cauliflower and Broccoli Gratin
- **Dessert:** Coconut Chia Seed Pudding

Day 11:
- **Breakfast:** Chia Seed Pudding Parfait
- **Snack:** Tomato Basil Bruschetta
- **Lunch:** Roasted Garlic Cauliflower Mash
- **Dinner:** Spaghetti Squash Primavera
- **Dessert:** Peach and Almond Yogurt Smoothie

Day 12:
- **Breakfast:** Avocado and Tomato Breakfast Toast

- **Snack:** Greek Yogurt and Berry Parfait
- **Lunch:** Baked Herb-Roasted Brussels Sprouts
- **Dinner:** Quinoa-Stuffed Bell Peppers
- **Dessert:** Strawberry Banana Oat Smoothie Bowl

Day 13:
- **Breakfast:** Chia Seed Pudding Parfait
- **Snack:** Crunchy Almond-Coconut Energy Bites
- **Lunch:** Eggplant and Tomato Bake
- **Dinner:** Crispy Baked Eggplant Parmesan
- **Dessert:** Cinnamon Baked Pears with Walnuts

Day 14:
- **Breakfast:** Avocado Toast Fiesta
- **Snack:** Savory Avocado Rice Cakes
- **Lunch:** Mushroom and Spinach Stuffed Bell Peppers
- **Dinner:** Cauliflower and Chickpea Curry
- **Dessert:** Peach and Basil Sorbet

Week 3

Day 15:
- **Breakfast:** Berry Blast Overnight Oats
- **Snack:** Crispy Roasted Chickpeas Trio

- **Lunch:** Mediterranean Chickpea Salad Bowl
- **Dinner:** Baked Lemon Herb Salmon with Roasted Vegetables
- **Dessert:** Cinnamon Baked Apples

Day 16:
- **Breakfast**: Egg White Veggie Scramble
- **Snack:** Zucchini Chips with Herbed Yogurt Dip
- **Lunch:** Salmon and Quinoa Stuffed Bell Peppers
- **Dinner:** Spaghetti Squash Primavera with Grilled Chicken
- **Dessert:** Coconut Berry Smoothie Bowl

Day 17:
- **Breakfast:** Greek Yogurt Parfait Delight
- **Snack:** Cheesy Cauliflower Popcorn Bites
- **Lunch:** Vegetarian Lentil Soup
- **Dinner:** Stir-Fried Tofu and Broccoli with Brown Rice
- **Dessert:** Baked Almond-Orange Ricotta Pancakes

Day 18:
- **Breakfast:** Quinoa Breakfast Bowl Bliss
- **Snack:** Avocado and Tomato Salsa with Baked Pita Chips

- **Lunch:** Citrusy Quinoa Salad with Grilled Chicken
- **Dinner:** Sweet Potato Crust with Mushroom and Spinach Quiche
- **Dessert:** Minty Watermelon Slush

Day 19:
- **Breakfast:** Sweet Potato Pancakes Extravaganza
- **Snack:** Sweet Potato and Kale Chips
- **Lunch:** Zesty Shrimp and Avocado Wrap
- **Dinner:** Lemon Herb Chicken Skewers with Quinoa Pilaf
- **Dessert:** Cocoa-Dusted Almonds

Day 20:
- **Breakfast:** Avocado Toast Fiesta
- **Snack:** Caprese Skewers with Balsamic Glaze
- **Lunch:** Veggie-Packed Minestrone Soup
- **Dinner:** Vegetarian Black Bean Enchiladas
- **Dessert:** Ginger-Turmeric Golden Milk Latte

Day 21:
- **Breakfast:** Chia Seed Pudding Paradise
- **Snack:** Edamame and Roasted Garlic Hummus
- **Lunch:** Feta Stuffed Chicken Breast and Spinach

- **Dinner:** Balsamic Glazed Salmon with Roasted Vegetables
- **Dessert:** Berry Chia Pudding Parfait

Week 4

Day 22:

- **Breakfast**: Spinach and Feta Omelette Fiesta
- **Snack:** Rosemary and Parmesan Chickpea Crunch
- **Lunch:** Turkey and Vegetable Skewers with Quinoa
- **Dinner:** Quinoa and Vegetable Stir-Fry with Tofu
- **Dessert:** Avocado Chocolate Mousse

Day 23:

- **Breakfast:** Spinach and Mushroom Omelette Roll
- **Snack:** Baked Sweet Potato Chips
- **Lunch:** Lemon Garlic Tilapia with Asparagus
- **Dinner:** Cauliflower and Broccoli Gratin
- **Dessert**: Greek Yogurt Parfait with Pistachios and Honey

Day 24:

- **Breakfast:** Sweet Potato Breakfast Hash
- **Snack:** Spicy Edamame Nibbles
- **Lunch:** Whole Wheat Spaghetti with Fresh Tomato Sauce

- **Dinner:** Mushroom and Spinach Stuffed Chicken Breast
- **Dessert:** Coconut Chia Seed Pudding

Day 25:
- **Breakfast:** Avocado Toast Fiesta
- **Snack:** Tomato Basil Bruschetta
- **Lunch:** Roasted Garlic Cauliflower Mash
- **Dinner:** Spaghetti Squash Primavera
- **Dessert:** Peach and Almond Yogurt Smoothie

Day 26:
- **Breakfast:** Avocado and Tomato Breakfast Toast
- **Snack:** Greek Yogurt and Berry Parfait
- **Lunch:** Baked Herb-Roasted Brussels Sprouts
- **Dinner:** Quinoa-Stuffed Bell Peppers
- **Dessert:** Strawberry Banana Oat Smoothie Bowl

Day 27:
- **Breakfast:** Chia Seed Pudding Parfait
- **Snack:** Crunchy Almond-Coconut Energy Bites
- **Lunch:** Eggplant and Tomato Bake
- **Dinner:** Crispy Baked Eggplant Parmesan
- **Dessert:** Cinnamon Baked Pears with Walnuts

Day 28:
- **Breakfast:** Quinoa Breakfast Bowl Bliss
- **Snack:** Savory Avocado Rice Cakes
- **Lunch:** Mushroom and Spinach Stuffed Bell Peppers
- **Dinner:** Cauliflower and Chickpea Curry
- **Dessert:** Peach and Basil Sorbet

Day 29:
- **Breakfast:** Berry Blast Overnight Oats
- **Snack:** Crispy Roasted Chickpeas Trio
- **Lunch:** Mediterranean Chickpea Salad Bowl
- **Dinner:** Baked Lemon Herb Salmon with Roasted Vegetables
- **Dessert:** Cinnamon Baked Apples

Day 30:
- **Breakfast:** Egg White Veggie Scramble
- **Snack:** Zucchini Chips with Herbed Yogurt Dip
- **Lunch:** Salmon and Quinoa Stuffed Bell Peppers
- **Dinner:** Spaghetti Squash Primavera with Grilled Chicken
- **Dessert:** Coconut Berry Smoothie Bowl

RECIPES INDEX

Your Daily Planner

Studies indicate that those who maintain a daily log of their food intake have significantly greater success in maintaining their health and reducing their weight compared to those who do not. Keep a journal of the renal diet recipes you attempt and the physical changes that occur in your body with this daily planner. This will not only give you an excellent summary of your development, but it will also serve as a useful guide for you going forward as you pursue your health goals.

DAYS	RENAL DIET RECIPES	REMARKS

How Did We Do?

Have you experimented with the recipes in our Renal Diet cookbook for Seniors? Did our recipes make managing your renal health easier and more delicious? We'd love to hear your thoughts. Please share your feedback with us. This is how we improve. Positive reviews and insights from wonderful customers like you, will help others feel confident about choosing this book and can guide those who are looking for a helpful resource to manage their renal health-related issues through healthy cooking.

Thank You and Happy Cooking!

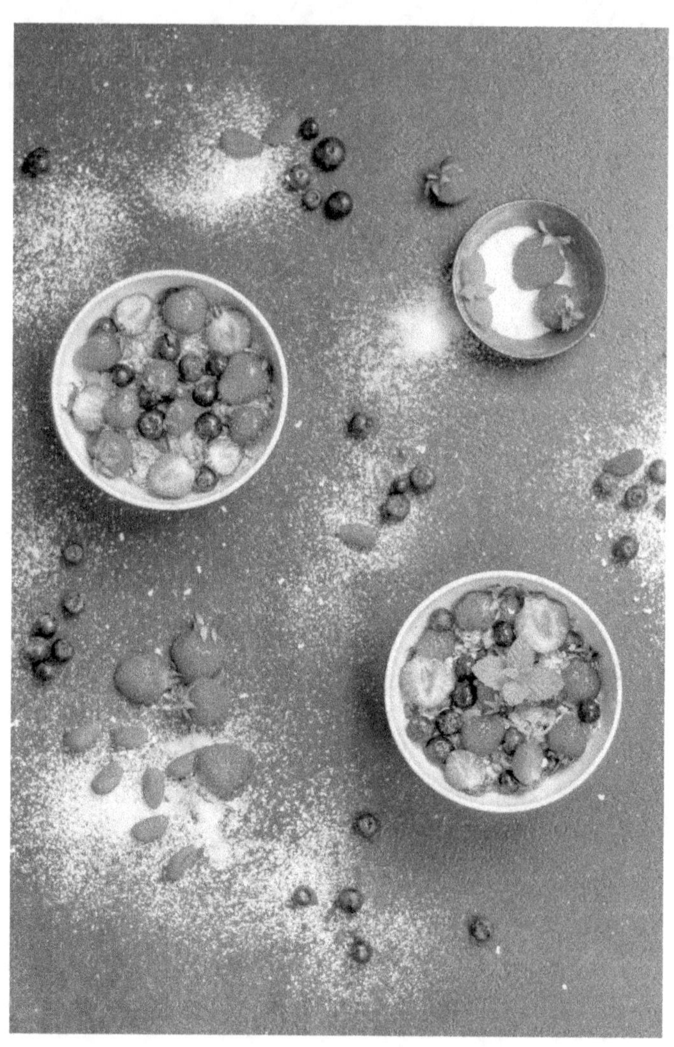